Mental Health Issues in Primary Care

Mental Health Issues in Primary Care:
A Practical Guide

ELIZABETH ARMSTRONG

MACMILLAN

© Elizabeth Armstrong 1995

First published 1995 by

MACMILLAN PRESS LTD
Houndmills, Basingstoke, Hampshire RG21 2XS
and London
Companies and representatives
throughout the world

ISBN 0–333–60675–2

A catalogue record for this book is available
from the British Library

10	9	8	7	6	5	4	3	2	1
04	03	02	01	00	99	98	97	96	95

Printed in Malaysia

CONTENTS

LIST OF FIGURES

Few people can fail to be surprised when they learn of the sheer enormity of the misery and costs experienced by the general population because of mental health problems, be they severe but rare illnesses such as schizophrenia, or the generally less severe but much more common depression and anxiety from which many if not all of us may suffer at some time in our lives. Surprised too, when they hear statistics such as the high proportion of people who commit suicide who have been to see their doctor in the week before their death. Mental illness can be treated and there is much that can be done to prevent suicides. The selection of mental illness as a key area in *The Health of the Nation* (1992) is helping to focus our attention on doing both.

Of all the health services, primary care is ideally placed to act. It has been known for more than a decade that over a third of all people consulting their general practitioner have psychological problems and that very few of these people are referred subsequently to psychiatric services. Mental health skills are, therefore, vital for all primary care professionals, as well as for specialists. However, much depression and anxiety still goes unnoticed in primary care, partly because it may masquerade as physical illness, and there is a clear need amongst primary care doctors and nurses for help in the detection and treatment of mental illness. Mrs Armstrong's book provides that help.

The book evolved from the Mental Health Facilitator Project, begun in co-operation with the Department of Health, and is a remarkable example of targeted research providing practical solutions within a short space of time. Although aimed at the nursing profession in primary care, it will be useful to a broader audience of doctors, other health professionals and managers who must all be involved in a co-ordinated approach to tackling mental illness in primary care settings. In addition to describing a wide range of mental health problems encountered in primary care and their diverse presentations, Mrs Armstrong discusses the treatments available and strategies for prevention.

Aiming to identify and treat effectively more mental health problems in primary care will not lead to extra work. The workload is already there, generated by the increased rates of consultations and referrals of people with an undiagnosed or poorly managed psychological disorder. On the contrary, better detection and management decreases that workload and has benefits for patients and professionals alike. This book will provide a resource for all those who wish to achieve these aims and I commend it as a major contribution to their efforts.

Dr Rachel Jenkins
Principal Medical Officer
Department of Health

PREFACE

When I began work on the Mental Health Facilitator Project in February 1991, it would have been difficult to foresee the enormous explosion of interest in mental health that there has been among nurses and doctors who work in primary care. Undoubtedly the inclusion of Mental Illness targets in the *Health of the Nation* strategy has been partly responsible, along with the Defeat Depression Campaign, jointly run by the Royal College of Psychiatrists and the Royal College of General Practitioners. Also contributing has been the increasing visibility of mentally ill homeless people on our streets – though in primary care terms this may be something of a red herring.

The difficulty remains that traditionally the focus of most health care in GP surgeries and clinics has been on physical illness. Typically, GPs eliminate the physical before considering the psychological. Practice nurses have taken their lead from this. The high profile given in the last 10 years to the prevention of heart disease and cancers has concentrated health promotion initiatives in these areas. There are indications that a substantial portion of this effort may be failing to meet the health care needs of a large number of those who consult GPs and nurses. Research has shown that as many as two-thirds or more of surgery attenders may be suffering from some level of psychiatric disorder. Much of this co-exists with physical illness, emphasising the interdependence of mind and body. Yet it is only the body which has received attention!

Health professionals are increasingly aware of the limitations of the traditional approach. They are also searching for practical ways to address their clients' psychosocial as well as physical health needs. The large number of requests that I receive asking for help in this area is testimony not only to the level of interest but also to the scarcity of reliable advice and information.

This book is designed to meet some of the needs. It is not a psychiatric textbook. Rather it is designed to help primary health care team members cope with some of the common mental health problems they meet every day. Inevitably there will be gaps – for which I apologise. This is a huge subject and we have to start somewhere.

The book is intended primarily for nurses – for practice nurses and other community nurses, for primary care facilitators and FHSA nurse advisers. There is much here for GPs too, and I hope it may be of use to health promotion officers and to FHSA managers. The vast majority of people with psychiatric illness are cared for in primary care. Most primary care professionals do not have specialist mental health qualifications but that they need mental health knowledge and skills is undeniable. By pointing to this need, and highlighting the gaps, this book may also serve to help purchasers and commissioning agencies make rational decisions about spending NHS money.

Above all, I hope this book is practical. I have tried throughout to draw attention to sources of helpful material: to books, literature and audiotapes for patients, educational programmes for professionals as well as organisations offering information and support in mental health related fields. Where full details are not given in the text, the Resources section at the end of the book will supply addresses.

To all those who have helped me tackle these issues over the past three years, whether or not your name is listed below, I should like to offer my thanks. In particular to the GPs, nurses, practice managers and staff of six practices in inner London. Thankyou for being my guinea pigs. Without you, none of this would have been possible.

EA
February 1994

I should like to thank all my colleagues on the research team and the steering group of the Mental Health Facilitator Project for their help and support during the life of the project and the writing of this book. Many other colleagues have contributed ideas and suggestions.

In particular, thanks are due to Dr Keith Lloyd for help in producing the flow-charts in Chapters 3 and 4; to Nicola, Elspeth and Hazel, and to Cathy and her colleagues for helping with the framework in Chapter 9; to Nicky, Karen and Doriette for their patience and endless checking of lists; and to Dr Andrew Craig for his help with Chapter 6.

Acknowledgements are due to Radcliffe Medical Press, Oxford for permission to print the table (Figure 3.1) in Chapter 3, and to Cathy Sutherland and Dr George Walker for information about the Bath Model Practice Project.

Finally, special thanks to Dr Rachel Jenkins for her encouragement to write this book, and for her many helpful suggestions; to Elaine Fullard for her support when the going got tough, and to my husband, who has lived with the book for the past year, and read the proofs.

CHAPTER ONE

Mental health and illness in primary care

AN UNCONSIDERED TRIFLE?

To most people – and that includes many health professionals – mental health means mental illness; mental health care means care of people with psychiatric, usually psychotic illness delivered by psychiatrists, psychologists, registered mental nurses and other specialists.

There is no dispute that seriously ill people need specialist care, but the majority of people with mental health problems do not have a psychosis. The most common mental illness is depression. Over 90% of mentally ill people are never referred to specialist care (Goldberg & Huxley 1980). They are treated by their GP. Or rather they go to their GP. Too often they are **not** treated.

THE SIZE OF THE PROBLEM

Almost one-fifth of the health service budget is spent annually on psychiatry. The total costs for neuroses in primary care are much higher than the costs for schizophrenia across all services. Psychiatric disorders are the third commonest reason for consultation in general practice after respiratory disorders and cardio-vascular conditions (Shah 1992).

Goldberg & Huxley (1980) have described a series of levels and filters (Figure 1.1) by which people with psychiatric illness obtain the care they require. Level One represents what seems to be the amount of psychiatric illness in the general population, though prevalence rates are by no means universally agreed.

The first filter is the decision of the individual to consult his/her GP – about one in four of the population will consult a doctor at some time in their lives for psychiatric reasons. It looks as though a majority of those with psychiatric illness do in fact seek medical help.

The second filter represents the recognition of the problem by the GP. A variety of research evidence suggests that GPs may detect as little as a third to a half of the psychiatric problems which present, though there are

1

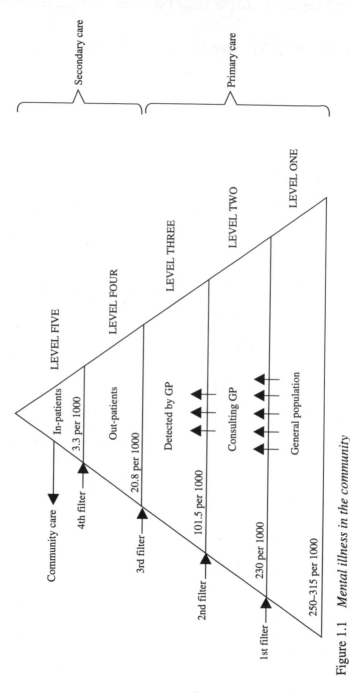

Figure 1.1 *Mental illness in the community*

Source: (Personal communication, Dr Rachel Jenkins, Department of Health) after Goldberg, D. & Huxley, P. (1980) *Menta Illness in the Community: The Pathway to Psychiatric Care*, Tavistock Publications

2

wide differences between practices and between individual GPs within a practice (Goldberg 1992). Level Three, then, is those who are detected – which also means those who have a chance of receiving appropriate care.

The first three levels and the first two filters illustrate the situation in primary care. The third filter is referral to psychiatric outpatients – and it is significant that only about 10% of patients are ever thus referred. In general those that are referred seem to be the most ill.

Levels Four (out-patients) and Five (in-patients) represent the secondary care services. Most people will eventually move out of hospital care back into the community. The majority of these will be people with chronic schizophrenia. Under the *Care Programme Approach* (DH 1990) which came into force in April 1991, all of these people should have a planned programme of care and a professional key worker from the specialist sector. They remain the responsibility of the secondary care services, though of course they will also have a GP. Good communication between GP and specialists will be essential to ensure optimum care.

But, what of the remaining 90%? The majority of this group is likely to be suffering from depression, anxiety or a mixture of the two. That is, non-psychotic illness. Such conditions are also sometimes called neuroses or affective (mood) disorders. Except for those who are seriously suicidal, there is no reason to suppose that they cannot be perfectly well cared for in general practice settings. For most people, going to see the GP is a completely acceptable thing to do. Going to a psychiatrist is much less so.

As Figure 1.1 illustrates, less than half of those people who consult their GP with psychiatric problems are recognised. Although Goldberg and Huxley's original work was published in 1980, recent figures suggest that little has changed. Results from audits conducted in a number of inner London GP practices taking part in the KCW FHSA Mental Health Facilitator Project (Chapter 2) were remarkably consistent with the published research. The audits used the 12-point Goldberg General Health Questionnaire (GHQ) (Goldberg & Williams 1988) to show that GPs were recognising at best nearly three-quarters of patients with psychiatric illness, but at worst less than a third. The GHQ is a well-validated research instrument which identifies 'psychiatric cases' not simply those who are feeling a little low or having a bad day. In some practices as many as 80% of consecutive attenders at surgery were 'positive' to the GHQ, depending on the threshold used. Not only were some of the GPs dismayed by their own low recognition, but the prevalence of illness was seen to represent a frighteningly large potential workload. GPs were already feeling that the workload was unmanageable.

3

In discussion, most seemed aware that a considerable proportion of their patients had psychological problems, but these problems were usually ascribed to social factors outside the GP's control. This apparently led some of the doctors to believe that because they can do nothing to influence the patient's social problems, neither can they do anything about the resultant depression. Yet it has been shown that recognition by the GP improves the outcome (Paykel & Priest 1992). In other words, those that are recognised get better more quickly than those who are not. In addition, depression reduces motivation. Treating the illness enables people to regain some control over their circumstances.

Particularly in inner cities, there is a plethora of helping agencies, statutory, voluntary and private, offering assistance to people with social, emotional and psychological difficulties of every kind. Counselling, for instance, has been shown to be effective with women suffering from acute or chronic depression and problems with a partner (Corney 1992). The reluctance of GPs to refer patients to such agencies – which was demonstrated in the audits described above – seems to have more to do with lack of knowledge than lack of agency.

Other negative attitudes were apparent. Most doctors felt that patients do not like being told they are suffering from depression and will not accept the diagnosis. Yet when the records of GHQ positive patients were reviewed, in less than a third was there any mention of a 'psychological' diagnosis in the preceding three months. Observations of actual consultations revealed little attempt to elicit depressive symptoms.

There appeared to be a marked reluctance on the part of most GPs to prescribe antidepressants. The main reasons for this seemed to be: (a) a belief that these drugs were not effective in 'reactive' depression, and (b) patients would not take them because of troublesome side effects and the perception that they are addictive. Yet antidepressants are known to be effective in moderate to severe depression and they are not addictive, unlike the benzodiazepines.

There was very little attempt to monitor people who were prescribed these drugs, or to offer them information and support. Nurses who could have taken on this responsibility were usually too busy with income-generating tasks like cervical cytology and immunisation. Such prescriptions as were given were usually for too small a dose and for too short a time (Paykel & Priest 1992).

These observations illustrate some of the ways in which the psychological needs of patients in the practices in this project were not being met. Experience from a parallel study in south-west England suggests that this is not a phenomenon confined to inner London.

4

PROFESSIONAL APPROACHES TO HEALTH AND ILLNESS

Doctors

The GP is both the beginning and the end of the health care system in Britain. The sick person goes to his/her GP for help and may receive medication there and then. Often the doctor will monitor the condition over more than one consultation before offering treatment.

Alternatively, the GP may refer the patient to a hospital specialist either for advice on appropriate treatment, or for hospital care. The consultant will eventually refer the patient back to the care of the GP.

The position of the GP is thus crucial. On the accuracy of the diagnosis depends not only appropriate treatment, but also the specialist to whom patient is referred.

Jenkins (1992a) shows that the fragmentation of medical specialties into separate organs and systems which happened at the end of the last century was responsible for the division of mind from body in medical theory. Yet it has been known from ancient times that mind and body are intimately linked. She considers that the one patient/one diagnosis model which has since dominated medical training fails to do justice to patients who have multiple difficulties.

A more multiaxial or multidimensional approach is advocated. While it is acknowledged that many GPs do take a holistic view of diagnosis and management, nevertheless the attitude that says 'if it isn't physical, it must be psychological' is still very common. Even where the links between mind and body are recognised, the attitude that if you take care of the physical, the psychological will take care of itself seems frequently to guide medical (and nursing) practice.

An illustration of this is seen in the antenatal patient who at 24 weeks has still not felt foetal movements. She is naturally referred back to the obstetrician, but although the appointment might be a week ahead, no attempt is made in the meanwhile to offer her support in what must be an intensely anxious wait. It does not occur to the GP that referral to the health visitor or midwife might be also be appropriate.

Many non-medical health care workers refer disparagingly to something they call the 'medical model' without always being clear what is meant by this. One aspect is undoubtedly the one patient/one diagnosis model described here.

The other major discredited feature seems to be the one consultation/one prescription reflex. In the study mentioned above, there was one GP who required the receptionist to place a blank prescription form in the top of the records of each person to be seen in surgery. It is still widely believed by doctors and nurses that many patients are not satisfied with a consultation unless they leave with a prescription.

A recently published study by van de Kar *et al.* (1992) in Holland suggests that a need for information rather than medical treatment is a significant determinant of the decision to consult the GP. The authors suggest that unnecessary consultations and 'waste of GP time' might be prevented by offering patients better information, for instance about the efficacy of medical care.

Nurses

For a number of years nurse training has taken health rather than illness as its starting point. Project 2000 courses take this approach further. But, once trained, nurses still tend to take their lead from doctors. While this applies less to health visitors and district nurses than hospital nurses, it is very much the case with practice nurses, many of whom go straight from hospital into general practice with no community nursing training or experience.

Less than half of practice nurses currently in post (Atkin & Lunt 1993) have attended a validated practice nursing course; only 12% are qualified as district nurses and even fewer (3%) as health visitors – though more than half undertake home visiting as well as surgery work. Moreover, practice nursing courses do not lead to a formally recognised community nursing qualification, which could well be a factor in the relatively low uptake of these courses, and which continues to be a source of considerable anger among profession leaders.

Continuing education for this group of nurses was, until relatively recently, difficult if not impossible to obtain. The work of primary care facilitators, FHSA nurse advisers and a number of active and committed practice nurses has changed this situation (see Chapter 2). The Royal College of Nursing's *Nursing Update* series of television programmes with regularly published linked supplements in *Nursing Standard* is a major advance in making educational material much more accessible to nurses who are isolated from the mainstream. A problem remains that television programmes are expensive to make, and sponsors are more readily found for subjects like nutrition and coronary heart disease than for depression and schizophrenia.

It has been left to a pharmaceutical company to provide the major mental health related training initiative for practice nurses. The suspicion is always there in such cases that the motive is more to increase the sales of a particular drug, than to provide education , however high quality the input.

Practice nurses are employed by GPs. Their roles and responsibilities are therefore defined largely by the GP whose knowledge of the scope of nursing practice may be limited. Indeed, the nurse may have been appointed specifically to increase practice remuneration through meeting cervical cytology and immunisation targets.

While this is a perfectly legitimate aim, too great a concentration on physical health targets can distort the nurse's care decisions. One nurse was observed persuading a recently arrived refugee to have a cervical smear. The woman had attended the practice to consult the GP about her two children's respiratory infections. As a new patient, she had been diverted to the nurse for a 'health check' with the result described. No attention was paid to her unkempt, harassed appearance, or to the fact that she was a refugee whose husband had remained at home in a war-torn city, although this was known. It needed very little imagination to understand that she was potentially depressed and obviously very anxious, yet little was done to ensure that she had appropriate support. Cervical cancer was likely to be very low on her scale of priorities at that point in her life.

The need to meet targets thus becomes the over-riding motivation for the health check, and no attempt is made to listen to the patient's own beliefs about her health or to give her the opportunity to express her own needs and wants.

'User empowerment' has become a cliché in talking about relationships between professionals and clients in health care. Essentially, what it means is that the client is guided in identifying his/her own health care needs. The professional provides information to enable the client to make informed decisions and choices about how to meet which needs.

This sounds fine in theory but in practice it can be threatening to professionals. Allowing clients/patients to make their own choices means allowing them to make the 'wrong' choice – and accepting it when they do!

THE POTENTIAL FOR PREVENTION

As long ago as 1981 the Royal College of General Practitioners published a report on the opportunities which exist for the prevention of psychiatric disorders in general practice. In the same year a similar report was published on the prevention of arterial disease.

The second report led to an explosion of activity. The prevention of heart disease has become a normal part of general practice work. Much effort is expended in making sure people have regular blood pressure and cholesterol checks. Patients are advised about their diet and helped to give up smoking on a routine basis.

The first report has disappeared almost without a trace. Heart disease is much more glamorous than depression. Prevention, though now perfectly respectable, is almost entirely devoted to physical illness.

The rationale behind the cardio-vascular disease report was that sufficient evidence existed to suggest that a high proportion of heart attacks and strokes were preventable if only current knowledge was applied in practice.

Newton (1992a) makes the following observation about mental illness: 'current knowledge is sufficiently impressive that we can at least begin to think about prevention and about how existing services might be influenced by . . . research.' There is a familiar ring to that statement.

We know a good deal about the factors which put people at risk of developing psychiatric illness. There is evidence that appropriate intervention with high risk groups and individuals at times of life transition or crisis might be preventive (Newton 1988).

It has been shown that depression has a better outcome if detected by the GP. Early detection leading to quicker and more effective treatment should therefore prevent more serious disorder (Goldberg 1992). Newton (1988) quotes a study by Wing and colleagues which suggested that advance preparation of schizophrenic patients for industrial placement could help prevent relapse. More research is needed to assess the effectiveness of such interventions though health visitors have been shown to be successful in both detecting and managing non-psychotic postnatal depression if suitably trained and using appropriate tools (Briscoe 1989, Holden *et al.* 1989).

The opportunities remain. The need for more research should not be used as an excuse to delay acting on the knowledge we already have.

PROMOTING MENTAL HEALTH

Newton (1992a) describes two models of prevention: one is the 'medical' model of targeting vulnerable individuals, a concept which will be further developed in Chapter 7; the other is the 'health promotion' model which 'targets the general population with measures known to be preventive of disorder for a few and assumed to be health-promoting for the rest'.

These two models are seen to co-exist and both have value particularly for heart disease where risk factors are widespread in the population, but where the majority of deaths will fall within the moderate to low-risk group simply because this group contains the largest number of people.

For mental illness the position may be reversed. For instance, most cases of depression are likely to fall within high-risk groups. Preventive activities are likely to be most effective if targeted at these groups. The same might be true of health promoting activities. An example might be organisations such as Homestart which aim to offer friendship and support to isolated mothers.

The antecedents of much mental ill-health are social, for example poverty, poor housing and unemployment. Health professionals do not have direct control over these factors. There are in any case many good reasons other than preventing mental illness for tackling these social ills – as Newton points out. There is, however, one area at least where population-directed health promotion measures might be valuable, and that is in reducing the stigma which still attaches to any form of mental illness.

Fear of madness is widespread and deep-rooted. Health professionals are not immune from this fear, and it may colour the responses made to people suffering mental distress. Fear may also be one reason why people often do not disclose their distress directly to the doctor, but may prefer to present with more acceptable physical symptoms. Turner (1986) describes a survey by Tyrer which reported that more than a third of patients preferred to see a psychiatrist at their GP surgery because there was less stigma attached. Turner suggested that as a first step it was the attitudes of doctors which needed to be changed. Doctors are still widely respected, and turned to for advice when matters of health are discussed.

HEALTH OF THE NATION

Mental health, and in particular untreated depression has been shown to be a major problem for primary care. The Government White Paper of 1992 *The Health of the Nation* acknowledges the size of this problem, and the human costs to individuals and families of mental illness in all its forms. It sets out a strategy for health in England and selects five key areas for action. One of these is mental illness.

National objectives and targets have been set, the achievement of which will mean real improvements in health which can be measured. It is acknowledged in the document that the paucity of morbidity data in this, as in other areas, makes the setting of measurable targets for the reduction of morbidity not yet possible. But while work goes on to develop suitable outcome indicators, two of the three main targets relate to a reduction in suicide rates. The third, unquantified at this stage, looks to an improvement in the health and social functioning of mentally ill people.

The Targets

'A. To improve significantly the health and social functioning of mentally ill people.

B. To reduce the overall suicide rate by at least 15% by the year 2000 (from 11.1 per 100 000 population in 1990 to no more than 9.4).

C. To reduce the suicide rate of severely mentally ill people by at least 33% by the year 2000 (from the estimate of 15% in 1990 to no more than 10%).'

Target A is intended initially to focus on the severely mentally ill with the possibility of being extended over time to include those less severely ill. There are responsibilities for primary care implicit in this target as well as more obviously for the secondary care services.

For instance, many people with chronic schizophrenia attend their GP surgery for regular injections of antipsychotic drugs – which will often be given by inexperienced practice nurses. Some of these patients will have lost contact with their specialists and may therefore be missing out on essential skilled rehabilitation, social care and support. People with chronic schizophrenia should have a written care programme with an identified care manager and named key worker (see Chapter 6). Auditing the care of these people within individual practices would reveal the numbers of patients involved, and identify both their unsatisfied needs and the training needs of practice staff.

Targets B and C can seem remote from the experience of many primary health care professionals. In a GP practice population of about 2500 there is likely to be only one death from suicide every three to four years (Wilkinson 1989). However, most people who kill themselves have been in contact with a health professional, usually a GP, shortly before. About 70% will be suffering from depression. A reduction in the overall suicide rate will therefore depend in large measure on better recognition and treatment of depression.

Deliberate self harm (or parasuicide) is much more common – about three to four cases per year on a list of 2500. About 10% of these people will eventually succeed in killing themselves.

Failed suicide attempts, for example drug overdoses are often unsympathetically treated in Accident and Emergency Units. Self-inflicted injury is viewed as less worthy of attention than a 'pure' accident. People may be offered no psychiatric assessment or follow-up and be discharged into the same situation which led to the incident (Evans 1993). Better follow-up care, perhaps by primary care staff and/or social workers, CPNs or psychologists may reduce the likelihood of a repeat, perhaps successful attempt, and help the patient learn more appropriate ways of coping with social difficulties.

CONCLUSION

It has been shown that the prevalence of mental disorders is high in primary care patients, yet traditionally most primary care professionals are more concerned with physical health problems. Dealing with psychological difficulties is seen as time-consuming. Giving patients opportunity and space to talk about their concerns rather than simply stating presenting symptoms is seen as 'opening the floodgates'. Doctors and nurses believe that they have no time to deal with the resultant deluge and feel they will be submerged.

These concerns, though real, are based more on myth than reality. It is perfectly possible to elicit the symptoms of depressive illness in a relatively short consultation if done in a systematic, focused way. Nor are doctors and nurses powerless to help. Effective treatments and management strategies do exist.

Patients, too, are aware of the constraints on the doctor's time. Collusion between doctor and patient, or nurse and patient, in concentrating on physical symptoms may give immediate satisfaction, but may not succeed in getting to the root of the problem. The inadequately treated patient is likely to return – again and again and again.

Spending time at the beginning to correctly identify the patient's problems and needs may actually result in saved time later. This is the pay-off for the primary care team. People who get better don't bother the doctor!

CHAPTER TWO

Facilitating change

Change is never easy. Changing time-honoured ways of providing care for distressed people is likely to be particularly threatening for doctors and nurses. People in health care like to think they are doing the best they can for their patients. Admitting the need for change is saying 'I could do better'. It can also feel like saying 'I've been getting it wrong'.

These two things are not the same. Recognising that in any endeavour there is always room for improvement opens the way to professional growth and development. It isn't that health care has been wrong up to now. Only that things are different. Perhaps the latest research has given new insights, making the old way of doing things seem less appropriate. Not recognising this can be a recipe for stagnation and complacency.

The pace of change in the Health Service in the last few years has been phenomenal, and many people believe that the changes have been forced through with little consultation. This has left many primary care doctors and nurses feeling that the only stable thing in a quicksand world is their clinical work with their patients – and even this is encroached upon by the ever-increasing demand for statistics and reports coming from FHSAs.

To be asked then to change aspects of clinical practice related to a subject in which most primary care workers have little formal training – mental health – can seem like the last straw.

THE KCW FHSA MENTAL HEALTH FACILITATOR PROJECT

It was in this maelstrom of change that the Mental Health Facilitator Project was set up in early 1991. It was funded by the Department of Health and supported by Kensington and Chelsea and Westminster Family Health Services Authority (KCW FHSA). The Project was designed to evaluate the role of a facilitator working with a group of inner London GP practices in the area administered by the FHSA and covered by what was then Parkside Health Authority.

The facilitator's main task was to help GPs and their staff consider how best to:

1. improve the early detection and prompt treatment of people with anxiety and depression;
2. devise ways of identifying and offering support to people at risk of these conditions (Jenkins 1992b).

The project was set up as a controlled trial involving a total of 18 GP practices. Initial evaluations were undertaken in 12 practices, following which 6 of them (the intervention practices) had the services of a facilitator for about 18 months. The second 6 practices were the controls and received no intervention. The final 6 practices, the control-controls, had only the final evaluation.

Since the aim of the project was to evaluate the facilitator's impact, it was necessary to account for the effects on the intervention practices of any outside influences. The evaluation alone could be responsible for raising awareness of the issues, hence the need for a third group of practices who would not have undergone the initial investigations.

The evaluation used measures of:

- GP recognition and management of, as well as attitudes to, depression and anxiety;
- use of resources by practices;
- patient outcome.

FACILITATORS – HISTORY AND BACKGROUND

Facilitators have been around in primary care for more than a decade. The idea is usually said to have started with Dr Arnold Elliot, an Islington GP, who was employed by North East Thames Regional Health Authority to visit other GPs to help them gain access to grants to improve their premises. It was thought that personal contact and help from a trusted colleague could be more effective in stimulating and promoting change than any number of official exhortations and directives which frequently remain unread (Allsop 1990).

The success of Elliot, and the publication in 1981 of the RCGP report on the prevention of cardio-vascular disease in general practice, prompted the major development of the facilitator role which is still going on.

In 1982 in response to the challenge posed by the RCGP report Elaine Fullard and her colleagues set up the Oxford Prevention of Heart Attack and Stroke Project. They aimed to introduce to general practitioners and

13

their staff a simple, opportunistic method of health screening which could identify people who were at risk of cardio-vascular disease. To help the participating practices introduce the screening system, and support them while they became accustomed to using it, the project used a facilitator who came from a background in nursing, health visiting and health education.

It is hard to credit now that when the Oxford Project began there was very little organised preventive or health promotion activity in general practice settings. Very few people had their blood pressure measured on a regular basis; even less had their smoking habits recorded or were actively helped to give up; and hardly any had their weight recorded or were given dietary advice unless they specifically asked for help with slimming. Even cervical cytology and immunisation were not necessarily seen as a major GP responsibility.

The achievements of the Oxford team have been well documented (Fullard *et al*. 1987) though most of the published work – and most of the criticism – has concentrated on the screening and audit methods which were used. For the present purpose the processes used by the facilitator to enable and encourage practices to take up the scheme, are more important than the scheme itself. The skills are transferable.

Just as in Elliot's earlier work it was personal contact between the facilitator and the practice teams on a regular basis which enabled the interventions to succeed.

The publication of the Oxford team's first report (Fullard *et al*. 1984) led to widespread interest in the potential of facilitators to influence change in general practice. Over the next few years a number of other facilitators were appointed, first within the Oxford region and then further afield. Appointments have continued to expand.

There are now well over 350 facilitators in post nationwide. They have formed a professional association (the Association of Primary Care Facilitators) which provides support, educational activities, bursaries and a newsletter. The Health Education Authority's Primary Health Care Unit houses the National Facilitator Development Project which continues to promote and advise on further appointments. An induction course for new facilitators is held twice a year and other courses are organised according to demand.

Facilitators are now a well established part of primary health care. For the majority of them their work is still mainly focused on the prevention of cardio-vascular disease with interest in related conditions such as diabetes. They help primary care teams develop their expertise in enabling patients to make life-style changes which would benefit their health. The Health of the Nation targets are central to this work.

14

FACILITATORS AND PRACTICE NURSES

When Elaine Fullard began her work only about 15% of GPs employed the full quota of ancillary staff for which they were entitled to reimbursement. There was therefore a great deal of scope for encouraging the employment of more practice nurses. Practice nurse numbers have expanded rapidly in the intervening years.

However, working in general practice can lead to professional isolation for nurses – as is so for GPs. Whereas GPs have for a long time had ways of gaining access to continuing education, until recently this has not been the case for practice nurses. GPs are actively encouraged to keep up to date by such devices as the post-graduate education allowance. No such incentive exists for nurses. At the time of writing the post-registration education and practice (PREP) proposals of the United Kingdom Central Council for Nursing, Midwifery and Health Visiting (UKCC) have still not been implemented after several years of waiting.

In addition GP employers may be ignorant about the scope of nursing practice and about different forms of nurse training. In a recently reported survey (Robinson *et al.* 1993) less than half the GP respondents saw lack of training opportunities as a hindrance to role expansion for practice nurses. Many GPs still seem to believe that training as a nurse, however many years ago and at whatever level, fits any nurse to work in whatever situation the employer chooses without further training. In today's complex health care such attitudes are frankly dangerous.

That this situation is now changing is largely due to the stimulation given to practice nursing by facilitators. Practice nursing used to be a backwater. It is now in the forefront of developments in primary care, and attracts high quality individuals. These nurses are no longer satisfied with poor educational opportunities, nor are they prepared to accept the less than ideal working conditions and remuneration which many of their number have endured in the past.

The growth in the appointment of practice nurse advisers by FHSAs is helping to improve the training and professional support offered to practice nurses. Many nurse advisers are former facilitators, and there is considerable overlap between the roles both in work done and skills required. The major distinction to be made seems to be that the nurse adviser concentrates on nurses, as the title implies. The facilitator, who is likely to have been appointed to achieve some specific change or to develop a particular project, will be working, in the main, with complete practice teams. In addition nurse advisers whose roles are based on those of their medical adviser colleagues may find that their main job is to provide nursing advice to the FHSA or purchasing authority rather than support for nurses in the field.

As Allsop (1990) has pointed out the facilitator is an agent of change, and may of necessity be a transitional figure. Once a particular change has happened the facilitator should no longer be needed. However, the skills of managing change are applicable in a variety of situations. The facilitator need not be confined to the prevention of heart disease – as many facilitators have demonstrated.

It was the aim of the KCW FHSA project described above to show that a facilitator's skills could be used to influence the way GPs recognise and manage depression and anxiety. Part of the facilitator's job was to produce a transferable model which would be of use to existing facilitators in primary care, to encourage an extension of their role into the field of mental health. It was not to create a whole new army of specialist facilitators.

MODELS OF FACILITATION

A brief description of the Oxford Prevention of Heart Attack and Stroke Project has already been given. The salient features of Fullard's model of facilitation may be summarised in the following four activities:

1. *Audit*. She used a baseline audit to answer the question 'How are we doing?' and to provide a point against which to measure progress. The screening method devised by the team was consistent with published research but it is easy to argue with research. Methodology can be criticised. You can say that the research does not apply in your situation because you are different. There are any number of excuses. It is much less easy to argue with the results of an audit undertaken in your own practice with your active participation.
2. *Protocols*. She advocated the use of simple protocols, for instance in blood-pressure measurement, so that each member of the practice was working to agreed standards. This helped the practice nurse, who had responsibility for the screening programme, know when she should refer to the GP for treatment decisions. It gave the nurse confidence that her referrals would be taken seriously by her GP colleagues. Working to agreed protocols also improves consistency of approach by GPs within the team.
3. *Resources*. She provided information and literature to practice nurses to back up the health advice they were giving to their patients. Where there was no practice nurse, she encouraged practices to employ one, and actively helped them through the process.
4. *Training*. She provided training for the whole practice team in recognition of cardio-vascular risk factors, and specific training for nurses

and other staff for their roles in the screening method. This included teaching receptionists to invite patients for health checks. The part receptionists play in 'selecting' the sort of care each patient receives is frequently overlooked. Yet even in their basic role of making appointments for patients they exercise considerable influence. Deciding which patient sees which doctor may help to determine the kind of treatment the patient receives.

Personal contact between facilitator and practice was an essential link in all these activities. Change would not have happened without this element.

The value of facilitator-assisted change has been clearly demonstrated by Dietrich and his colleagues (1992) in the United States. These researchers used a randomised trial to compare the effects of two interventions, alone and in combination, on the implementation into community (GP) practice of measures designed to increase the early detection and prevention of cancers.

The intervention which combined physician education with facilitator-assisted changes in practice organisation and service delivery produced the greatest improvements. Physician education alone produced only minimal changes.

The researchers concluded that facilitators are a useful resource for improving preventive and early detection services and could be used in other clinical areas – 'whatever the specific . . . services, a facilitator can improve performance'.

It is worth noting from this study that the facilitators were particularly concerned with helping the practices implement new systems for service provision. They involved the whole practice team in discussions and decision-making. They also provided a wide variety of tools such as record cards, flow-charts, protocols, health education leaflets and posters and patient-held diaries. Practices were able to choose which tools best suited their purposes. As in Fullard's model, the facilitators acted as a resource for the practice team. They were not there to see patients themselves.

Cockburn et al. (1992) report a study from Australia which compared three different approaches to marketing a smoking cessation kit to GPs. Although those doctors who received their kits from educational facilitators, as opposed to couriers or through the post, were shown to have been much more likely to use it, the researchers concluded that the differences were not significant enough to justify the greatly increased cost of using the facilitator approach.

This result seems to argue that facilitators should not be used simply as a marketing tool. The facilitators in this case saw each GP on only two occasions over a 6-week period. Most British facilitators would regard this as far too short a period over which to demonstrate effective change. An intervention using fewer facilitators, each supporting more GPs over a longer time-scale, might have produced more cost-effective and significant use of the kit.

A group from Southampton (Spiegal *et al.* 1992) have described a model for managing change in general practice which is based on ideas from industry. They suggest a sequence for action which includes the following components:

1. *An assessment of the practice.*
   Is the practice ready for change?
   Who will help and who will hinder?
   Who are the key people?
2. *Negotiation.*
   How to get agreement for change.
3. *Designing and Implementing the change.*
4. *Review.*
   How well did we do?
5. *Celebrating success.*

This group advocates a highly structured approach to getting started on the business of change which may seem unnecessarily time consuming and bureaucratic. However, as they point out, taking time at the beginning to get the basics right is likely to save a great deal of time later, and be less costly in the long run.

There is an important message here for facilitators who are often under pressure to produce results unreasonably quickly because of short term contracts. Change which happens superficially with inadequate groundwork will not stick. This is a waste of time and effort. It also discredits the change.

An illustration is provided by the introduction of health promotion clinics into general practice following the 1990 contract. They proliferated fast, in an ill-thought-out way which resulted in blatant abuse of the system. The whole idea of health promotion in general practice has suffered as a result.

Another important message from the Southampton group was that change happens most easily where there are slack resources. There is relevance here for the KCW project since in central London primary care is stretched to almost intolerable limits and, as the *Tomlinson Report* (1992) pointed out, is underdeveloped compared with other regions of the country. The scope for real change was therefore always going to be small. The project offered the facilitator's help as the only 'extra', when what really seemed to be needed was more people on the ground to cope with the enormous workload. This is of course hindsight.

The approaches to facilitating change as described above have common elements. Pringle *et al.* (1991) describe the process as an exercise in navigation. Their three basic questions summarise it neatly:

1. Where are you now?
2. Where do you want to get to?
3. How are you going to get there?

The facilitator can be either an external agent or someone from within the practice. The internal facilitator of change, perhaps a practice nurse, may have certain advantages in knowing the practice, the personalities involved and the best way to present the change to maximise its chances of being taken up.

The external facilitator has the advantage of no preconceived notions about the practice, and can bring in good ideas from elsewhere. Individual practices vary enormously and those who work in general practice are often isolated fom their peers. The facilitator working with a variety of practices and across professional boundaries can encourage the exchange of information and strategies.

FACILITATING CHANGE IN MENTAL HEALTH

In deciding the approaches to be used in the KCW Project, all of the above-mentioned sources, and others, contributed ideas. The model, although originally developed for use in mental health is, like all facilitator models, readily adaptable to a variety of situations. The model and its practical applications can be described thus:

It has been called the **GARTER** model (Figure 2.1) from the initial letters of its key words. This is apt, for the overall aim of the facilitator is to support the practice in making changes to the way it meets the needs of its patients.

The process should be a continuous one. At the Review stage of the cycle there will be indications of the need for further change – but at this point much of the groundwork will not need to be repeated.

Groundwork

Laying the foundations of a successful project is vital, and should not be rushed, whatever the pressures. Setting up meetings in GP practices takes time. The first step should be a letter to the senior partner, but this will need to be followed up fairly swiftly by a phone call to the practice manager. It is

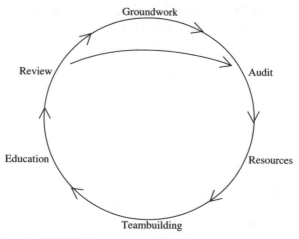

Figure 2.1 *GARTER – a model for facilitating change*

worth waiting until as many of the practice team as possible are available. Visiting staff individually is extremely time-consuming and repetitive, but may have to be done in those few practices which still have no regular meetings. Two things are of prime importance:

1. A clear statement about the change which is to be advocated. Research evidence should be available showing that such a change would be of benefit to patients. There should also be some benefit, some pay-off, for the practice which needs to be explicit from the start. It is well worth taking the time to prepare an introductory information package for practices – but it should be short and to the point.
2. A non-threatening approach towards getting to know the practice and its internal dynamics. The aim is to encourage the team to reflect on the topic in question, to decide for themselves what the needs of their patients are in this area, and to look at the way they currently meet the needs. It is not to insist that they change in any particular way.

The danger here is that the team will take a totally different view of the problem from that taken by the facilitator. Some compromise may be necessary in order to build up trust within the practice. Can some of their worries be tackled without jeopardising the facilitator's ultimate aims?

A possible way of getting to know how a practice works is for the facilitator to spend time during the working day with every member of the practice team including sitting in on GP consultations. This is presented to the team as 'Getting to know what you're up against'. Additional aims would be to build up relationships with possible allies and identify areas where suggestions for change might be acceptable and not too disruptive. Possible blocks will also become apparent: the partner who has no interest in mental health; or the practice which feels that because it has one psychotherapy session per week, it has solved all its patients' difficulties.

This activity is not without its dangers particularly within the GP consultation. Clear boundaries to the facilitator's role need to be set:

(a) Confidentiality must be preserved, not only for the patient, but also for the GP. The facilitator is an observer, not a judge and is not there as a spy for the FHSA.
(b) The facilitator's presence in the consulting room must be acceptable to the patient. Each patient should be asked.

The facilitator may observe something which seems inappropriate. As an example consider the young mother who expresses suicidal ideas in front of her unruly child. This is not taken seriously by the doctor. As a guest in the practice, the facilitator must resist the urge to intervene.

Staying silent during such an encounter may be very stressful, but it would be unethical to appear to disagree with a doctor in front of the patient. It may be possible to discuss the issue with the doctor afterwards, but not all doctors will respond positively to perceived criticism from a non-medical person. The facilitator will need to have in place a good personal support system to help handle such difficulties before exposure to this kind of risk.

Ideally, the impetus for the next step should come from the practice rather than the facilitator, but this may or may not be feasible, depending on the sophistication of the practice team.

Audit

The main aims of the audit are to answer three basic questions:

1. What is it like now?
2. How would we like it to be?
3. How can we make it better?

Answering these questions involves gathering data about a particular issue; agreeing on the required standards and deciding on the necessary processes to achieve the standards. Data from the initial investigation will provide a baseline against which progress can be measured. This is essential for effective review (Pringle *et al.* 1991).

At best a practice should design and conduct its own audits. Given the high work-load in primary care it may help if the facilitator has a ready-designed protocol and offers to conduct an audit personally.

The audit is a quality exercise. It is not research. It involves measuring actual performance against a standard which has been set and agreed by the practice team. Provided the team is fully involved and committed to the audit, ideally with the support of the local medical audit advisory group (MAAG), it should present no threat.

In the KCW study the GPs were denied feedback from the research team following the initial evaluation. The audit was designed partly to fill this gap. It was conducted by the facilitator, who personally gave the results to the doctors. As in the research protocol, the 12-point Goldberg GHQ (Goldberg & Williams 1988) was used to measure the ability of the GPs to recognise potentially depressed patients, but the scores were calculated on a practice basis rather than for individual GPs. This was to avoid introducing an element of competition which could have been destructive of some already fragile partnerships.

The audit also made an assessment of the care received by GHQ positive patients (those with a level of psychiatric disorder) over the preceding 3 months. Details of the audit protocol are in the appendix.

There are many other possibilities for mental health related audits:

1. What are the criteria used for the prescribing of benzodiazepines? How many long-term users do you have?
2. Antidepressant prescribing; are they prescribed in therapeutic doses? How long for? Are they monitored? How good is patient compliance?
3. How many patients with long-term mental illness do you have? Do they all have a care programme in place? Do you know the name of the key worker in each instance?
4. How many attempted suicides have there been in the last year? Have all these people been offered appropriate follow-up support?

The audit results may be written up and presented as a short report for the practice. They will suggest areas for change but should not be used to fuel destructive criticism. The above examples could lead to plans for:

1. Devising a programme of tranquilliser withdrawal for long-term users.
2. Developing a system for close monitoring and support of people taking antidepressants.
3. Arranging a series of meetings with local community psychiatric nurses to develop closer working links.

4. Liaising with the local Accident and Emergency Unit to devise ways of ensuring better follow-up support for people who deliberately harm themselves.

Gathering baseline data and measuring progress may not be the only reasons for the audit. At the beginning of the KCW project, chronic schizophrenia and the short-comings of the psychiatric services dominated most doctors' thinking. Depression was on nobody's agenda. By highlighting the numbers of attenders in surgery who had psychological problems – the majority of whom were likely to be depressed – the audit was able to re-focus the discussion on the much more common problem. Perceptions were changed. Depression was clearly seen for the major issue it is.

Resources

If the audit gives the impetus for change, it also leads to further questions:

(a) What have we got that we can use?
(b) What else do we need?

There are a number of factors which come under this heading:

1. *People*. This might mean looking for extra nursing time perhaps to start a system for monitoring antidepressant usage, employing a counsellor or both. It might also mean looking to arranging sessional help from outside specialists, for example a social worker or clinical psychologist.
2. *Information*. Practices need information in a variety of forms: a detailed knowledge of local services, statutory and voluntary; literature for patients; posters for surgery displays; a practice library which will not only contain books and journals for the practice team, but also items which may be loaned to patients such as books or relaxation tapes.
3. *Tools*. This includes such things as agreed protocols and guidelines for the management of common conditions like depression and anxiety; screening questionnaires; guidelines for referral between different professionals and agencies and procedures for monitoring prescriptions.

Team building

Many people working in primary care see addressing their patients' mental health needs as opening a 'Pandora's box'. They say that they do not have the time to listen to people's problems. They have no confidence in their ability to help and they already feel so overwhelmed that there is no room to take on anything 'extra'. It is difficult to convince GP and nurse alike that recognising and caring for depressed people thoroughly is not adding extra work. It is coping better with what is already there.

No one person in the primary care team can do this alone. Today's health care, with its emphasis on prevention, health promotion and risk factor management is a complex business. The old model of one or two GPs with a couple of receptionists operating from a lock-up surgery with maybe a few hours a week from a practice nurse who doubles as secretary is less and less able to cope. This type of practice is still all too common in our inner cities. They are not necessarily 'bad' practices, but they cannot handle the increasing demands and expectations of patients.

As practices get larger and encompass more and more people from different professional backgrounds, it becomes vital for people to work together to define common goals and understand each other's roles and contributions. Failure to do this leads to much frustration, wasted time and duplication of effort – which costs money (Pritchard & Pritchard 1992).

Nowhere is this more apparent than in mental health care where effective help for people involves psychological, social and self-help measures as well as pharmacological treatment. With an average case-load of 300–600 depressed people, even the most dedicated GP could not hope to do more than scratch the surface without support, help and expertise from a variety of other sources.

Looking at the way the practice team itself functions is a first step towards building a unit which is confident that it can meet the needs of those who come for help.

Education

Most professionals who work in primary care are not mental health specialists. Many will discover that they need new knowledge and skills to improve their confidence and allay their fears. The facilitator can help by identifying sources of training.

Until relatively recently there was little available for primary care team members. The Defeat Depression Campaign, set up by the Royal College of Psychiatrists in association with the Royal College of General Practitioners is helping to change that by producing packs for both trainee and established GPs. The work of Gask and others (1992) has shown that GPs can learn effective psychiatric interviewing and problem solving skills relatively easily using video and audio feedback techniques. The skills learned persist over time.

Such training, known as problem-based interviewing, is also being adapted for practice nurses (Usherwood 1993b).

The Royal College of General Practitioners, in association with the Department of Health, the Mental Health Foundation and the Gatsby Trust has appointed an Educational Fellow in Mental Health in General Practice, one of whose key aims is the dissemination of knowledge to regional advisers and GP tutors – a cascade approach (Jenkins 1992b).

The Royal College of Nursing, supported by the Defeat Depression Campaign, has produced a mental health module in its *Nursing Update* continuing education series for nurses. The module consists of two half-hour programmes on 'Depression: Lifting the Cloud' and 'Suicide: A Target for Health'. The programmes were supported by written material published in *Nursing Standard* (Usherwood 1993a and Evans 1993), and can be seen at a series of RCN viewing centres around the country. A further module in the series plans to look at counselling skills.

A team-based course in primary mental health care is being developed by a group supported by the Royal Institute of Public Health and Hygiene.

Local resources should not be overlooked. Community psychiatric nurses could be a valuable source of expertise for their practice nurse colleagues, particularly in the care of people with chronic schizophrenia (Chapter 6).

Review

This activity serves a number of functions. It answers the question 'Have we achieved what we set out to achieve?' Thus it enables the practice to celebrate success, which is vital. We should always allow ourselves the well-earned reward. And it can offer a new baseline for further change.

The review is best done in the form of a repeat audit. It is at this stage in the process that the value of a well-conducted and well-written-up initial audit becomes apparent. Baseline figures will be available for comparison.

It is possible that the result will not to be as good as was hoped. Not everything planned has been achieved. A consideration of the whole process will identify the reasons why this might have happened. Perhaps the plan was too ambitious. If so, lessons can be learned for the next attempt at change – take things in smaller steps. Perhaps not everyone in the team was wholeheartedly behind the change. What could be done next time to ensure better support?

Even if the results fall short of expectations, something will have been gained. This should be recognised. But as achievement is applauded, complacency should be avoided. It is only by maintaining an atmosphere of reflective practice that beneficial changes can occur and go on occuring.

The model does not include a specific point at which change should be implemented. Rather, as new skills are learned and new resources acquired they should be used. In this way change happens naturally, without threat and in a way which causes the least disruption to the day-to-day work of the practice. It will be explicit though, and it will be recognisable in the results of the audit and review process.

CHAPTER THREE

Depression – cause and recognition

WHAT IS DEPRESSION?

Wilkinson (1989) defines depression as 'a persistant exaggeration of the everyday feelings that accompany sadness'. It is a disturbance of mood, of variable severity and duration, that is frequently recurrent and accompanied by a variety of physical and mental symptoms involving 'thinking, drive and judgement'.

It may be described as a continuum from a normal low mood which everyone experiences from time to time to a severe psychiatric disorder. (Paykel & Priest 1992).

It is important to distinguish 'feeling depressed' from 'having depression'. Clinical depression is a specific syndrome whose symptoms can be elicited. It isn't just a matter of having an off day or being unhappy. Nor should patients be labelled depressed just because their symptoms do not fit neatly into a common physical diagnosis (Wright 1988).

Dorothy Rowe, a psychologist who has written a number of books on depression for the general public, also stresses the difference between being unhappy and being depressed. She describes depression as 'a prison which we build for ourselves'. She goes on to say, though, that 'just as we build it for ourselves, so we can unlock the door and let ourselves out' (Rowe 1983).

Depression is common across cultures. In many languages there is no exact translation of the word depression. This should not be taken to mean that there is no experience of depressive illness.

During an audit in one of the practices in the KCW study the GHQ was completed by a non-English speaking Arab man with the aid of his wife, a fluent English speaker. The man was a refugee who had suffered a gun-shot wound some 2 years previously. This injury was still causing him considerable pain and disability. As she handed back the completed questionnaire to the facilitator, the wife expressed amazement at the feelings that her husband had talked about. She said 'I am his wife, and

27

I never knew he felt so bad'. Nor had his distress been recognised by his GP.

Recently, a group of Asian women discussed their experiences of depression on BBC Radio 4's *Woman's Hour*. They described it as 'the thinking illness', an 'illness of sorrow'. They were trapped inside 'these four walls'. They were very sad and couldn't laugh any more. They felt they were being punished for doing something wrong. The images they were using to illustrate their feelings were substantially similar to those that might have been used by an indigenous white woman. They will be familiar to anyone who has suffered from depression.

Depression is the most frequently occurring of all psychiatric disorders and the commonest seen in primary care settings. It is so common that it has been called the 'psychiatric common cold', but this should not imply that depression is always a mild condition. On the contrary, people do die from it. Most people who kill themselves are depressed. Reduction in suicide rates is a key mental illness target in the *Health of the Nation* strategy. One vital way to prevent suicide is to recognise and treat depression.

Prevalence

Estimates of the prevalence of depressive illness vary widely and will depend on the criteria used to define the condition. Paykel and Priest, in the consensus statement from the Defeat Depression Campaign (1992) suggest that the prevalence of major depression in the population at any one time is about 5% – but it is also suggested that as many as one person in three may experience an episode of depression during the course of their lives. About 5% of those consulting their GP will be suffering from major depression, another 5% will have milder symptoms, with a further 10% showing some distress.

These authors consider that at least one patient with mild depression or worse is likely to present at each GP surgery session. They also point to the research evidence which shows that in about a half of these patients, their depression will not be recognised.

Depression occurs at all ages, but tends to be more common with increasing age. It is not uncommon in childhood, and Williams (1993) draws attention to the large numbers of young people whose problems go unrecognised and untreated .

It is twice as common in women as in men, the reasons for which are unclear. There are suggestions that women may find it easier to talk about their psychological distress than men, and therefore be more likely to receive a psychiatric diagnosis. Men are said to be

28

more likely to resort to alcohol. There may actually be more depressive illness among women than among men, perhaps related to the social pressures of combining family and work responsibilities. Feminists may see the excess as being more to do with a power imbalance between female patient and male doctor, and with stereotypical attitudes of what constitutes a mentally healthy woman (Corob 1987).

Classification of depression

There are a variety of ways which have been used to classify depression. To non-specialists the most familiar are probably those of neurotic and psychotic depression, and of reactive and endogenous conditions.

Neurosis and psychosis refer to particular groups of symptoms, the main distinction being that neurotic depression does not include delusions or hallucinations (Wilkinson, 1989). The word neurotic in this context is a technical term. It does not imply attention seeking or complaining behaviour (Mann 1992).

Reactive depression suggests an illness which has arisen in response to a particular life event such as bereavement. This kind of illness is often regarded as understandable, almost normal. In consequence there may be a tendency to believe that treatment is not required, or will be ineffective. In contrast, depression which is said to be endogenous, that is arising spontaneously for no obvious reason, is considered to be amenable to treatment. Blacker and Clare (1987) state that very few episodes of depression arise completely out of the blue. The distinction is now thought outdated, and should not be used as a criterion for deciding on treatment.

Jenkins and Shepherd (1983) contend that many psychiatric disorders are associated with social, family and relationship difficulties, and can only be understood in this context. It has also been shown that outcome is closely related to social stresses and the quality of the patient's social support (Mann et al. 1981).

A further commonly seen classification is that of unipolar and bipolar depression. The latter is characterised by extreme mood swings from depression to mania. This is also known as manic depression or manic depressive psychosis, though these terms are sometimes said to be less acceptable to patients than bipolar depression. That may be so but it is interesting to note that the major voluntary organisation supporting these people calls itself the Manic Depressive Fellowship.

Unipolar depression refers to depression which occurs alone without manic episodes.

29

If this were not sufficiently confusing to the non-specialist, depression and anxiety are also often known as affective disorders, which simply means disorders of mood, or affect.

Causes of depression

There have been many attempts to discover the antecedents of depression. Psychological, biological and social factors have all been cited, but no single cause has been found nor is any single model entirely satisfactory in explaining how the condition arises. Newton (1988) surveys the literature in detail.

Psychological

Ideas of loss seem to be central, but it is not as simple as saying that bereaved people become depressed. Clearly many don't. Psychoanalytic theory suggests that the loss is of a kind which threatens self-esteem causing anger against the self, and helplessness.

Other psychological approaches also suggest a role for helplessness and a tendency to negative ways of viewing the world and events. Childhood environment and loss are seen as the origins of a learned sense of being a loser. People who believe themselves to be unable to exercise any control over what happens to them are seen as vulnerable to depression. This idea may seem familiar to those who are conversant with the concept of 'locus of control' in health (Niven 1989).

Biological

Research into possible biological causes for depression centres on genetics (is depression inherited?) and on physiological disturbances. There is good evidence for a strong inherited component in bipolar disorders and for some familial element, though less strong, in severe unipolar depression. A family history of depression is an acknowledged risk factor (Wilkinson 1989).

Physiological effects can follow life events. Alterations in brain chemicals such as the neurotransmitters serotonin and norepinephrine may occur. Reductions in the levels of these substances can cause disturbances of sleep, appetite, motivation and pleasure, all of which are symptoms of depressive illness.

The exact role played by such changes in the aetiology of depression is still unclear. Antidepressant drugs are believed to correct some imbalances but their mode of action is not always well understood.

Depression and physical illness

Depressive symptoms are a feature of a number of physical illnesses. Figure 3.1 summarises those that are considered to be causes, but depression may also complicate any life-threatening, disabling and painful illness. It can follow major surgery, particularly mutilating surgery for malignancies. It is common in people whose physical disabilities tend to lead to social isolation, especially those with hearing and/or visual impairment.

Social

In their classic study of working class women, Brown and Harris (1978) describe major life events and difficulties as 'provoking agents', but these events alone are not sufficient to cause depression. Nor are the effects of such events always additive – people suffering more than one such event are not necessarily more likely to become depressed. These authors consider that it is the meaning these events have for the individual, rather than the events themselves, which may influence whether or not the person becomes ill.

Moreover factors other than major events are also at work. These are referred to as 'vulnerability factors'. In the case of the working class women whom they studied, four factors are suggested:

1. Loss of mother before the age of 11.
2. Three or more children under 14 at home.
3. Lack of a confiding relationship, for example with husband or partner.
4. Lack of employment outside the home.

A third set of factors associated with symptom formation is also described. These include a severe event occurring after the onset of the illness, any past loss and a history of previous illness.

Torkington (1991) argues that in the case of black people in Britain, racism is a further, though rarely mentioned, factor in the development of mental illness. It is not simply that cultural ignorance on the part of health workers leads to misdiagnosis of black people as mentally ill, though this is important. It is rather that black people experience on a day-to-day basis a society which has deeply ingrained beliefs in the superiority of white cultural norms. This fact of black life is in itself debilitating. It is quite easy to understand that it could be responsible for a lowering of self-esteem. As Newton (1988) shows, low self-esteem is believed to be a factor in the development of depressive illness by many authors and researchers.

31

Neurological diseases	Parkinson's disease Multiple sclerosis Stroke Epilepsy Dementia
Malignant diseases	Lung cancer Brain tumours Cancer of the pancreas
Endocrine diseases	Hypothyroidism Cushing's syndrome Addison's disease
Kidney disease	Kidney failure Kidney dialysis
Anaemia	Iron deficiency Folate deficiency Vitamin B12 deficiency
Infections	Influenza Hepatitis Glandular fever Brucellosis Shingles
Side effects of drug treatment	Methyldopa Corticosteroids L-dopa Diuretics Barbiturates Reserpine
Drug withdrawal	Benzodiazepine tranquillisers Amphetamines Alcohol

Figure 3.1   *Physical causes of depression*
Source: Wilkinson, D.G. (1989) *Depression: Recognition and Treatment in General Practice*. Oxford, Radcliffe Medical Press.

Jenkins (1992c) has summarised current thinking on causes and aetiology. She describes the factors involved as:

1. Predisposing.
2. Precipitating.
3. Maintaining.

Each of these may have biological, social and psychological components.

1. *Predisposing factors* increase vulnerability. They may include heredity or physical damage such as birth trauma; emotional deprivation in childhood or a lack of a supportive relationship; and low self-esteem or learned helplessness.
2. *Precipitating factors* are those which determine the starting point of the illness. They may include disabling injury or malignant disease; recent major life events such as bereavement; and, in psychological terms, inappropriate responses to these events.
3. *Maintaining factors* prolong the illness and delay recovery. Examples might be chronic pain and disability especially sensory loss such as visual or hearing problems; chronic stresses involving personal and family relationships (lack of a supporting relationship being particularly significant), housing, work and finance and low self-esteem.

The recurring themes which clearly stand out are low self-esteem, loss (especially where a threat is involved) and lack of social support.

The costs of depression

Unrecognised and untreated depression has costs for both practice and patient.

The practice

Many doctors and nurses in primary health care express reluctance to improve their recognition of depressed people. There are a number of reasons for this, the main one being fear. Fear of the unknown, for instance:

- 'If we actively try to diagnose more depression, we won't be able to cope with the increased workload'.

On the face of it this might seem a reasonable enough reaction – except that recognition improves outcome (Jenkins 1992c). In other words those that are recognised get better more quickly than those who are not. It is well documented that in general practice people with psychiatric illness consult their doctors more frequently than others (Wright 1988). Evidence from the KCW study, and a parallel study in Bath (the Bath Model Practice Project – personal communication) confirms previous findings. Recognising and treating depression should therefore, over the longer term, reduce consultation rates and workload.

- 'If I ask people about their problems, the floodgates will open and I won't be able to cope.'

It may seem odd but in reality the floodgates don't often open, and if they do, most professionals cope very well. Nurses taking part in a recent pilot study which involved identifying people potentially at risk of becoming depressed (Chapter 7) did not usually have difficulties in keeping interviews to the point. Where people did want time to talk, most nurses were able to find time to listen, and they regarded this a good use of their time.

Techniques can be learned for eliciting the symptoms of depression within a normal consultation; of controlling the length of an interview while still allowing the patient/client space to express needs and concerns; and of negotiating with the patient an appropriate programme of treatment (Gask 1992).

If recognising depression takes time, not recognising it takes even more time. Furthermore, poor quality always costs money, often because an inadequately performed task will have to be repeated. It is expensive to do things badly. This applies as much to the business of health care as to any other business.

Data on the economic costs of depressive illness in primary care are sparse (Shah 1992), but the implications are that there is much scope for cost reduction. Undoubtedly one aspect is more effective use of antidepressants. An audit is likely to reveal that prescriptions are frequently given in sub-therapeutic doses and for too short a time, with minimal information to the patient and even less follow-up. Compliance with drug therapy is notoriously poor.

Better information combined with closer support and monitoring, perhaps by appropriately trained practice nurses may be able to improve this situation. A pilot study reported by Wilkinson et al. (1993) suggested that nurses were at least as effective as doctors in providing support. A larger scale study is now underway.

For the individual GP and practice, the clear implication of this seems to be that appropriate prescribing in adequate doses will increase the antidepressant drugs bill. Whilst this may be true, it is pointless to prescribe drugs in doses which do not work. There may also be a balancing effect in that there will be less prescribing of other drugs such as benzodiazepines, and fewer unnecessary hospital investigations ordered.

In overall Health Service terms prescribing drugs which no one takes or which do not improve patient outcome is a serious waste of scarce resources.

The patient

The consequence for patients of unrecognised and untreated depression can be devastating. They include increased risk of suicide and para-suicide; marital breakdown; and occupational problems such as increased sickness absence, inability to keep a job, difficulties over relationships with colleagues, decreased performance and increased risk of accidents.

For the children of depressed parents there may be increased risk of abuse. They are also vulnerable to emotional and learning difficulties which can predispose to mental illness in later life as well as limiting their ability to achieve their full potential.

Chronic non-psychotic illnesses such as depression, phobias and tranquilliser dependency lead to immense personal distress, suffering and lowered quality of life. They may trigger alcohol and drug abuse. They are a considerable burden on health services and lead to loss of productive capacity (Jenkins 1992c).

RECOGNISING DEPRESSION

There is said to be some measure of psychological component in up to a third of all general practice consultations. Awareness of the possibility of depressive illness therefore needs to be high on the agenda of all primary care workers.

In some situations, use of a screening questionnaire may be justified. One such situation is postnatal depression which affects 10% to 15% of all mothers. This is much higher than the rate for depression in the general population. Some health visitors use the Edinburgh Postnatal Depression Scale with all mothers at the routine developmental assessment carried out for babies at about six weeks of age (Cox *et al.* 1987). The 12-point GHQ is an alternative method of screening, though this instrument is not specific for depression.

Many mothers with postnatal depression remain untreated. Briscoe (1989) suggests that a large proportion do not actively seek help for their problems but their illness may have long term consequences for themselves and their families. Sharp (1992) suggests that one reason why postnatal depression is not always taken seriously by professionals is that it is almost entirely a general practice disorder. It is rarely seen in hospital psychiatry but this does not mean that it is not highly distressing and disabling.

Screening tools may also be useful in detecting depression in elderly people. Depression is common in old age. It should not be dismissed as part of the natural ageing process, and it needs to be distinguished from dementia. Depression is treatable and therefore well worth recognising.

GPs are required by their contracts to offer an annual health check to all patients on their lists over the age of 75 years. In fact most such assessments are probably carried out by nurses. Protocols and guidelines used should include assessments of mental state, both cognitive and memory function and screening for depression. A report published by the research unit of the Royal College of Physicians and the British Geriatrics Society (1992) suggests scales which could be used.

In everyday consultations a simple, open question such as 'How are you feeling in yourself?' could be used to provide clues as to whether a further assessment of mood is required. A systematic way of following up an answer suggestive of low mood is demonstrated in Figure 3.2. A series of more direct questions is used to elicit the major symptoms of depression.

Figure 3.2 is the first in a series of five information sheets ('depression cards') developed for the KCW study. The complete set was intended as an educational tool for use by the facilitator with the project GPs. It was also found helpful by nurses. The information is based on published sources including the consensus statement of a committee of the Royal College of General Practitioners and Royal College of Psychiatrists produced for the Defeat Depression Campaign (Paykel & Priest 1992) and the Effective Health Care Bulletin: The Treatment of Depression in Primary Care, from the School of Public Health, Leeds University (1993).

Nurses often comment that they are not taken seriously by GPs when they refer patients whom they think may be depressed. Use of tools like this could enable a coherent list of symptoms to be given, enhancing credibility. If drawn up and agreed by the whole practice team they could also provide a consistency of approach with benefits for more efficient patient care.

The questions (Figure 3.2) were used to distinguish between three levels of depressive symptoms, since this was found to be of most practical use.

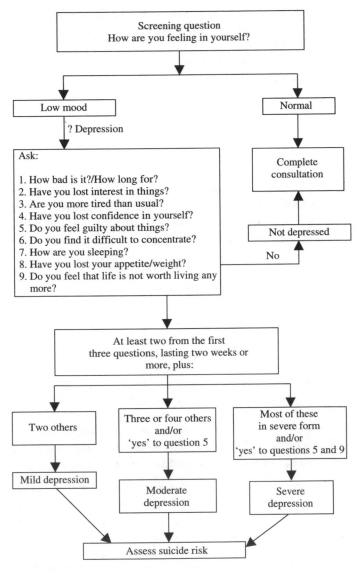

Figure 3.2 *Recognising depression*

In mild depression, the patient is usually distressed by the symptoms and has some difficulty with ordinary work and social activities.

In moderate depression there will usually be much more difficulty in continuing normal social, work and domestic responsibilities, and some symptoms may be marked.

The severely depressed patient will usually show considerable distress. Prominent among symptoms will be loss of self-esteem and feelings of guilt and uselessness. The full range of symptoms are normally present and the patient is unable to continue with his/her usual activities.

Problems in recognition

Use of tools already described may help to enhance detection skills, but lack of knowledge about depression is not only the reason for widespread non-recognition. It seems useful to divide the factors affecting recognition into those relating to the patient and those relating to the doctor, whilst acknowledging that the consultation is an interactive process in which either party can influence the other and therefore the outcome.

The patient

It has been shown that those who are not recognised have just as many symptoms as those who are and that their prognosis is not necessarily better. They are just as ill. The main distinguishing feature of the two groups seems to be that those who are not recognised are more likely to present with predominantly physical symptoms. They will not reveal their psychological distress unless specifically asked (Goldberg & Huxley 1980). These patients are often known as 'somatisers'.

Somatisation has been extensively researched and reported in the literature. There are a number of aspects worthy of note:

- Some people may perceive psychological distress in terms of physical symptoms, either because depression may make a pre-existing symptom worse or because people who are depressed frequently become excessively aware of bodily functions and sensations.
- There is a tendency to believe that doctors are only interested in physical symptoms. The physical symptom is an acceptable 'passport' to care. Doctors can seem to be busy people with little time to listen to problems. A presenting pain for which the cure is a pill may be seen as a way of getting some help without being perceived as a nuisance.
- A further factor is stigma. Psychiatric illness is still widely held to indicate weakness or poor character – views which may be held by

doctor as well as patient, and can be communicated in the course of a consultation to the detriment of appropriate care (Sims 1993).

Throughout the literature there are suggestions that people from non-white ethnic minority communities are more likely to present with somatic symptoms than indigenous British people. This belief may be misleading in that many white people also present with physical problems, although they may not be the same kind of problems (Mumford *et al.* 1991).

There is a need for much more research in this area before somatisation can be cited as a particular reason for non-recognition in black and Asian patients (Lloyd 1992). More importantly there may be a cultural mismatch between patient and professional. There are strong indications that if appropriate questions are asked in the patient's own language by a skilled and culturally well-informed doctor or nurse, then the nature of any psychological disorder will become apparent regardless of the ethnic background of the patient.

In practices whose population includes people from just one or two dominant ethnic groups, it should be the responsibility of at least one member of the primary care team to establish links with local community leaders and to learn something about widely held health beliefs within the community. This knowledge can be shared at team meetings so that the whole practice becomes more open to differences of approach. Patients will then be less likely to be labelled as 'problems' or 'inadequate' just because their behaviour does not conform to the accepted cultural norms of the staff (Mares *et al.* 1985). It is also less likely that they will become victims of unhelpful generalisations such as 'our Indian patients don't want to leave unless they've got a prescription in their hands'.

The doctor

Patients who go to their doctor with physical symptoms are normally examined appropriately. Treatment will be prescribed on the basis of the symptoms and further investigations may be ordered. Such a consultation may be satisfying to both doctor and patient. The presenting symptom has been taken seriously and dealt with, but it may fail to get to the root of the problem. Taking medicine which may temporarily relieve the symptom will mean that neither doctor nor patient need face the necessity of reviewing personal and social difficulties. There is unspoken collusion between the two to avoid distress.

Doctors who miss diagnosing depression may do so because they do not know how to manage it (Goldberg 1992). You don't ask the questions if you can't handle the answers.

Doctors who do detect depression have been shown to use well recognised behaviour in their interviewing style. There is nothing mysterious about these skills. They are useful to nurses as well as doctors. They include:

1. Making good eye contact with the patient from the start of the interview, and maintaining it – which means not looking at, or writing in, the records during the consultation. The patient remains the focus of attention.
2. Being able to clarify the complaint. This means listening to what the patient has to say and repeating it back (reflecting or paraphrasing) until the reason for consultation is clear. Verbal and non-verbal clues are important, and may be missed if full attention is not given to the patient both with ears and eyes.
3. Being able to ask appropriate questions in the right way. This not only means being familiar with the actual questions (Figure 3.2) but knowing when to use open questions and when to be more direct.

Nurses sometimes believe that asking closed questions – those which require only a 'yes' or 'no' answer – is wrong in most situations. This is not so. Open questions, such as: 'How do you feel about...?' or 'What do you think about....?' which require a more descriptive answer are useful for opening up the consultation, and providing the clues to things which are troubling the patient. Making a diagnosis, or eliciting symptoms needs more directive questioning, but it is important that questioning is relevant to the cues given. Such an interview can go on to negotiating and agreeing a management strategy with the patient.

Gask and her colleagues (1992) have devised ways of teaching psychiatric interview skills to general practitioners, skills which have been shown to persist over time. A training package for GPs based on Gask's work has been produced by the Defeat Depression Campaign and is available through local GP tutors.

The model used is known as 'Problem Based Interviewing' (PBI), and it is adapted for nursing use by Usherwood and colleagues at Rockingham College in Yorkshire (Usherwood 1993b).

Suicide

Suicidal thoughts can occur at any stage of a depressive illness. Depressed patients should always be assessed for suicide risk. As with recognition of depression a systematic approach is beneficial. The flow-chart (Figure 3.3) uses four indicators to assess the presence of risk, and its relative strength.

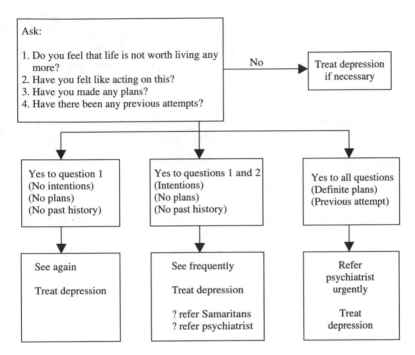

Figure 3.3 *Assessment of suicide risk*

- The presence of suicidal ideas in the absence of any intention to act, definite plans or a previous history would indicate a low relative risk, but would mean that the depression required active treatment. A nurse should always refer to the GP a patient who expresses suicidal ideas.
- Intentions, suggested by a positive response to the first two questions, indicate a moderate level of risk. The patient will need close supervision in the early weeks of treatment for depression, par-ticularly if antidepressants are prescribed. Some doctors say that anti-depressant therapy, which improves motivation, might actually temporarily increase the risk of suicide, as the previously lethargic patient gains the energy to act on his/her intentions.
- A positive response to the first three questions indicates a severe suicide risk and usually requires immediate referral for psychiatric

help. This is especially so where there is a history of previous attempts.

There are two further points which are worth mentioning:

1. It is not true that people who talk about suicide don't do it. They do. Expression of suicidal ideas should always be taken seriously.
2. It is not true that asking people about suicidal thoughts will 'put the idea into their heads'. On the contrary, affording people the opportunity to express these ideas and feelings can give considerable relief (Russell & Hersov 1983).

Finally, depression is a very common illness. The fact that it is so common leads some doctors to question its standing as a medical phenomenon – 'If it is so common, isn't it normal?'

Brown and Harris (1978) consider that this is a confusion of two separate issues. They contend that it is not logical to relate the frequency of a condition to its medical or non-medical status. They further state that the fact that depression and unhappiness overlap 'does not prevent them from being logically distinct concepts'.

Depression has been seen to be worth recognising for a variety of reasons, not least that recognition itself improves outcome. It is a treatable illness, the consequences of which, if untreated, can be devastating for individuals, families and society.

CHAPTER FOUR

Depression – options for treatment

Depression is a treatable illness. Many depressed people will recover spontaneously, but this is not a reason for dismissing the illness as of no consequence. Nor is it a justification for denying patients the care which could significantly shorten the period of their distress and improve their quality of life.

It is widely accepted that non-recognised or poorly treated patients are more likely to suffer chronic ill-health. A large number of authors have emphasised how painful, physically and psychologically, depression can be.

According to Wright (1993) managing depression well can be very satisfying for the general practitioner. It could be equally satisfying for the nurse to participate in a carefully thought-out practice protocol for the care of these patients.

MEDICAL AND NURSING APPROACHES TO CARE

Doctors traditionally talk about the 'clinical management' of a condition. Treatment is determined by diagnosis. The individual needs of the patient may be considered, but only in relation to the illness, and only the particular illness which has been diagnosed.

Nursing has more to do with meeting the health care needs of people. A particular medical condition is only part of the picture and it is the person who comes first.

Nurses are used to devising nursing care plans which work alongside and enhance medical care. Doctors sometimes seem to have little understanding of nursing approaches. That the nurse may have anything distinctive and different to offer patients is largely overlooked. It is even said by some that the nurse represents an unwelcome intrusion into the very special doctor/patient relationship.

This is clearly nonsense, particularly when caring for people with psychological and emotional disorders. The complexity of the issues involved, and the variety of options for care and treatment which exist

	Mild depression	Moderate depression	Severe depression
General	Acknowledge See again	Acknowledge See regularly	Acknowledge See frequently See family ? Refer psychiatrist
Psychological	?Counselling	Counselling or cognitive therapy (either in-house or use external agency)	
Pharmacological	None	Antidepressants plus information and monitoring	
Social	?Assess social difficulties ?Refer local agency	Assess social difficulties and refer to appropriate agency for help Does family need support?	
Physical	Depression in the presence of physical illness should be treated in the same way as depression without physical illness		
Self-help	Give suitable literature e.g. RCPsych leaflet 'Depression' Give advice on exercise, sleep, diet, problem solving, relaxation techniques as appropriate		

Figure 4.1   *Treatment options: summary*

make a multidisciplinary, team approach essential. The options are described under six headings and a summary is provided in Figure 4.1.

GENERAL

Recognition improves outcome but recognition is not enough if it is not shared with the patient. Acknowledgement is also vital.

Patients need straightforward explanations of the meaning of their symptoms. This might almost amount to 'giving the patient permission' to be depressed. Essential messages to convey are that depression is an illness with defined symptoms like any other illness. It will get better, though this may take time. It might help some patients to know that throughout their treatment a nurse will be available for support and advice should it be needed.

When referring a patient who may be depressed to the doctor, the nurse can begin to develop the necessary understanding and acceptance. Some depressed people feel they are 'going mad'. Reassurance that they are not is very important. Many patients will find considerable relief in such explanations.

It may help to relate the depression to a recent life event but care must be taken not to assume that because depression is understandable, it therefore does not require specific treatment.

There are some patients who will not accept a diagnosis of depression, whatever explanation is offered. Such patients present a difficult problem to doctor and nurse. Careful negotiations may be needed to achieve appropriate care. Understanding the patient's health beliefs is important. People who feel listened to and valued will gradually be able to relate physical symptoms to an illness which 'makes you more sensitive to pain than normal' (Wright 1993).

Even if the illness seems mild (Chapter 3) it will probably be necessary to see the patient at least once more, and an assessment of suicide risk should be made. A low risk of suicide may still be an indication for actively treating the depression, even though the patient may have no actual intentions to harm her/himself, no plans have been made and there is no previous history of suicide attempts.

More severe depression will require more frequent contact. Particular care will be needed if there is a greater risk of suicide, for instance if active plans have been made. It may also be necessary to see the patient's family to enlist their support and understanding, particularly if the patient is a mother with young children. The health visitor's assistance may be needed. Health visitors have wide knowledge of sources of support for parents within their local community. This knowledge is often overlooked by general practice colleagues especially in inner city areas where the health visitor may not be GP-attached. Referral to psychiatric services may need to be considered if the diagnosis is uncertain, if there appear to be psychotic features, or where there are serious concurrent conditions such as alcoholism or anorexia.

Severe suicide risk, where there is clear expressed intention, definite plans have been made and where there is a history of previous attempts, requires urgent referral to the psychiatrist. Compulsory admission to hospital under the Mental Health Act (Chapter 6) may be necessary (Tredgold & Wolff 1984).

For people whose illness does not require hospital admission, help may be provided by the Samaritans. This organisation offers telephone counselling 24 hours a day for people in despair. Their number should be easily accessible in all general practice settings. A supply of cards with the information can be readily obtained from local branches.

PSYCHOLOGICAL

Two main psychological methods are usually described: counselling and cognitive therapy. The Effective Health Care Bulletin (1993) considers that whereas there is evidence for the efficacy of the latter, more research will be needed before counselling can be confidently recommended. Many counsellors would consider that there is ample evidence of their effectiveness. A survey carried out for the Defeat Depression Campaign (MORI 1992) showed that the general public saw counselling as the most appropriate treatment for depression.

Counselling

Counselling has been described as 'the skilled and principled use of relationships to help the client develop self-knowledge, emotional acceptance and growth, and personal resources'. Among other things, it may help the client identify and solve problems or cope with difficulties in personal relationships, life transitions or crises (Rowland 1992).

Professional counselling by a trained counsellor must be distinguished from the use of certain core 'counselling' skills by other professionals. Such skills might include listening, reflecting and empathy. Basic communication methods like these are taught to nurses and doctors – and many other professionals. They may be used in the context of any patient contact to enhance the caring relationship.

The difference in professional counselling is that they are used as part of an ethical process to help the client learn to deal more effectively with his/her problems.

Counselling is not giving advice. Doctors and nurses are often consulted by patients as experts, for the knowledge that they have. They are expected to give advice. It may therefore be very difficult for them to also act as counsellor, since the relationships between doctor and/or nurse and patient and between counsellor and client are fundamentally different (McLeod 1992).

A major problem for counsellors, and would be employers, is that there is no universally accepted definition of what a counsellor is. There is no statutory body as there is for nurses or doctors. Currently anyone

46

can call themselves a counsellor after a minimum of training – or none at all.

The British Association for Counselling has an accreditation scheme which lays down minimum standards for the training and supervision of counsellors. Accredited counsellors are expected to conform to a published code of ethics and practice. There is a complaints procedure which can lead to expulsion of members who breach the code, but relatively few counsellors belong to this scheme though it is becoming a recognised and accepted standard (BAC 1990).

Employing a counsellor

The diversity of types of counselling, training courses and theoretical approaches makes it very hard for the GP to decide whom to employ. BAC accreditation provides a starting point. The BAC's Counselling in Medical Settings division produces guidelines to help (BAC 1993).

Unfortunately few current counselling courses train counsellors to work in primary care (source: Counselling in Primary Care Trust). Many counsellors have very little knowledge of medical terminology or of health promotion. This situation should improve within the next few years. Meanwhile, great care needs to be exercised in recruiting, lest GP and counsellor find themselves totally unable to communicate or understand each other.

The theoretical approach of the counsellor is important. Most counselling courses concentrate on one model, usually either the person-centred method of Carl Rogers (Rogerian Counselling) or the more practical problem-solving model of Gerard Egan. There are suggestions that the latter, with its emphasis on helping clients clarify goals and plan action, may be more appropriate for primary care (Morrell 1992). Experienced primary care counsellors often offer clients an explicit contract of a fixed number of sessions (say six). People who require more than this are no longer thought suitable for primary care therapy.

A particular difficulty can arise concerning drug therapy. Many counsellors believe that this prevents clients from benefiting from the counselling process. Antidepressants are said to present fewer problems than benzodiazepines or anti-psychotics, but counsellor and GP will need to agree an appropriate policy on drug use to avoid the possibility of conflict (Hammersley & Beeley 1992). It may be best to use antidepressants first, and commence counselling only when the mood begins to lift (Wright 1993).

Confidentiality is another potential source of conflict. In private practice, counsellors are accustomed to offering clients complete confidentiality. The GP, as referer, may not be comfortable with this, and in medical settings it may be inappropriate, especially if the counsellor learns something which is relevant to the care being provided by another team member.

A concept of team confidentiality may work better. Here the client is made aware at the outset that information may be shared with another member of the team unless the client specifically asks otherwise. If this is unacceptable, referral to an outside agency may be more appropriate.

The counsellor should understand that ultimate responsibility for the care of the patient in the practice rests with the GP. Good systems for communication between counsellor, GP and other team members are an essential part of working together. Communication doesn't just happen. It needs planning. Protected time should be set aside for regular meetings.

Practical aspects of employing a counsellor also need to be considered. The most important are availability of a quiet, undisturbed room and suitable remuneration. The use of volunteer counsellors in NHS premises seems undesirable. They will either be poorly trained and inadequate for the job, or their professional skills will be undervalued by the paid members of the practice team.

Trained counsellors are expected to have regular supervision. This provides support for the counsellor and is an essential component of professional counselling because of the stressful nature of the job. Therefore supervision time must be allowed for in the counsellor's working hours.

Effectiveness

Whether or not counselling is effective is a fundamental question which still needs to have a definitive answer. Corney (1992a) considers that recent studies of counselling with specific client groups do tend to give support to its value in general practice. There are however suggestions that some people may be harmed by counselling. It does not benefit everybody. The wide variety of theoretical approaches used make it important to find out which ones work. It is also important to know what level of skill the counsellor needs for advantage to ensue.

BAC accreditation is seen as a basic qualification by many in counselling. Further training is said to be needed for primary care work. This represents a very expensive and lengthy process. It is important to consider whether lower levels of skill might be equally effective. There is evidence that other professionals, trained in counselling skills, can be successful with some client groups.

The classic case is the study by Holden and her colleagues (1989) of counselling by health visitors. These authors showed that health visitors who had been given short training in Rogerian techniques could improve the outcome for mothers with postnatal depression.

Corney (1992b) suggests ways in which evaluation could be built into the ongoing work of the counsellor and the practice. Regular audits might provide another method of testing effectiveness. Important points to be clear about are:

1. What it is you want to measure?
2. What information do you need?
3. What is the best (and easiest) way to get the information?
4. Keep it simple – audit doesn't have to be research.

Kiernan (1992), a GP in inner London, showed that provided the patient demonstrated commitment to therapy, there was a reduction in GP consultation rate and in drug use once therapy was completed. Commitment could be improved if waiting time to see the counsellor was as short as possible, and if the GP spent some time preparing the patient for therapy. The increased workload implied by this preparation was felt to be justified by the results (personal communication).

Cognitive therapy

Cognitive therapy, also known as cognitive-behavioural therapy, is a fairly recent psychological technique for treating depression developed by Beck and colleagues in the USA.

Cognitive techniques have been shown to be effective in some types of depression and are thought to reduce the likelihood of relapse (Paykel & Priest 1992). An examination of available evidence for the Effective Health Care Bulletin (1993) concluded that cognitive therapy was as effective as the 'treatment normally received in primary care' but there were problems in interpreting the research because not all studies use the same outcome measures. More research is needed. There does seem to be a consensus that this kind of treatment might be usefully combined with antidepressants (Sheldon et al. 1993). It may be a treatment of choice for patients who refuse drugs.

The availability of cognitive-behavioural therapy is very variable. The techniques may be used by clinical psychologists employed by health authorities or trusts. Many of these will take direct referrals from GPs, and in some cases self-referral by patients.

There are problems with access to all types of psychological treatment in the NHS. In some instances this is because there are simply too few therapists to cope with the demand. Waiting lists tend to be long. Many centres will offer initial assessments within two or three weeks but it may take several months before a full course of treatment can be arranged. This is unacceptable to depressed people and their GPs.

Some patients arrive in therapy via psychiatric outpatients. Unnecessary appointments and time-wasting might be avoided if better communication existed between the various therapies and local GP practices enabling more appropriate referrals to be made from the beginning. Some counsellors may offer cognitive therapy.

In the cognitive theory of depression, a 'triad' of negatives is described:

1. A negative perception of self – 'I'm useless'.
2. A negative interpretation of experiences – 'Nothing good ever happens to me'.
3. A negative view of the future – 'It'll never get any better' (Wilkinson 1989).

Intrusive, negative 'automatic' thoughts concerned with low self-esteem, self-blame and self-criticism are present. Learning to identify and challenge these thoughts is central to treatment.

Other features of treatment are helping the patient learn to correct thinking errors such as 'all or nothing thinking' (I forgot Judy's birth-day. I must be a rotten husband); 'overgeneralising' (Nothing ever goes right for me); and learning to recognise unhelpful attitudes which have arisen from past experience.

A full course of treatment provided by a psychologist may last between 15 and 30 hours. France and Robson (1986) believe that many of the techniques of cognitive therapy could be learned by GPs and nurses and used in primary care settings. The simple methods they describe do not demand long sessions, and could be provided over a series of short appointments. Most of the work will be done by the patient between visits to the surgery.

In addition these authors consider that, particularly with the mild depression which is very common in primary care, elements of the techniques could be used alone, without necessarily having to provide a full course. In particular, they suggest that 'thought spotting' and correction are valuable.

Initially, the patient is asked to keep a record of negative automatic thoughts. Once he/she has learned to recognise them, and the feelings associated with them, they can then be challenged and answered. The Beck Depression Inventory is used to measure progress. France and Robson (1986) give details of all of these methods and others in their book *Behaviour Therapy in Primary Care: A Practical Guide.*

Other psychological therapies

There are at least as many psychotherapies as there are types of counselling. Distinctions between them are often far from clear (Howard 1992). Labels may be different. Techniques are very similar.

As with counselling, there is no statutory regulatory body for psychotherapists. Those who practise within the NHS will usually also be doctors, nurses, psychologists or social workers. Outside the NHS, anyone can practise as a psychotherapist. As with counselling, there is no legal requirement for any kind of training. This makes it extremely confusing for doctors to find sources of reliable therapy for their patients, and for patients to know that their therapist is reputable. There are some professional organisations such as the British Association for Psychotherapy. In general it would seem wise to advise patients to ensure that any private therapist they consult is a member of a recognised body.

Maxwell (1990) gives a useful overview of the types of therapy available from the NHS, from psychodynamic psychotherapy to everyday psychotherapeutic techniques which may be used by any health professional from GP to practice nurse. The latter are mainly the communication skills already described, especially listening and hearing what has been said – characterised by one psychiatrist as 'listening with your ears open'.

Although many psychotherapists would consider that they were successful in treating depressed patients, their small numbers, and the length of time taken for treatment – years in some cases – make most of these therapies second-line strategies rather than suitable methods for primary care settings.

PHARMACOLOGICAL

The main drug treatment for depression is antidepressants. These drugs have been shown to be effective in moderate to severe depression provided they are given in therapeutic dose for an adequate period. They are effective regardless of the cause of the illness. Decisions about drug therapy therefore need to be made on the basis of severity. Antidepressants may not be effective in mild depression (Wilkinson 1989, Effective Health Care 1993).

They are not addictive (Paykel & Priest 1992). The fact that they are often perceived to be so by both the general public and some professionals may be due to confusion with the benzodiazepines. The latter are certainly habit forming. Some benzodiazepines have in the past been prescribed as a treatment for depression. They are now considered best reserved for short-term uses, especially in severe disabling anxiety (Chapter 5).

Types of antidepressant

1. The tricyclics

This group of drugs has been available in general practice for more than 30 years. They are tried and tested and their side-effects are known. They have been shown to be effective in moderate to severe depression and are relatively cheap.

There is a wide range of such drugs available. The most commonly used are amitriptyline (Tryptizol, Lentizol), imipramine (Tofranil) and dothiepin (Prothiaden). All antidepressants are equally effective in relieving symptoms. The differences lie mainly in side-effect profile and toxicity, and are generally small in spite of manufacturers' claims (Lacey 1991).

It is usual with the tricyclics to begin treatment with a low dose and to increase over a week or two to the therapeutic level, which, in the case of amitriptylline will be 125 to 150 mg a day. Doses lower than 75 mg a day are not effective (Paykel & Priest 1992).

The antidepressant effect takes 2 to 3 weeks to develop, but side-effects are likely to be felt quickly. These are commonly anticholinergic effects such as dry mouth, constipation, urinary retention and blurred vision. Sedation may also be a problem, though since these drugs have a long half-life, they may be taken in once-a-day doses. The patient may be advised to take his/her dose in the evening, when the sedative effect could be beneficial. Alternatively, a less sedative drug such as nortriptylline (Allegron, Aventyl) may be tried (Crammer & Heine 1991).

Tricyclics need to be used with care in patients with heart disease or epilepsy. They are very toxic in overdose, and their use in suicide is well documented (Effective Health Care 1993). For this reason, great care needs to be exercised when prescribing these drugs for patients who express suicidal thoughts. Careful monitoring and close support of patients in the early weeks of treatment should reduce this risk.

This might also improve patient compliance with antidepressant treatment, which is notoriously poor. It is wasteful and pointless to prescribe drugs for patients which they will not take but there are ways in which this situation might be improved. They can be summarised as Agreement, Information and Support:

(a) Agreement
    The decision to prescribe antidepressants should be a joint one between patient and doctor. Ideally it should be part of a 'treatment package' in which the patient is a full participant. It does not seem unreasonable to explain to patients that drugs are expensive, and that while the doctor is happy to prescribe what is needed, the

patient also has a responsibility to take what is prescribed. Patients cannot expect their medication to help them if either the prescription is not dispensed or the tablets stay in the bathroom cabinet.

If the patient does not agree to take the medicine as prescribed, then perhaps medication is an inappropriate treatment for that patient. Alternative strategies need to be discussed. Treatment should be negotiated with the patient, not imposed through a 'doctor knows best' attitude.

(b) Information

In order to give informed consent to treatment, patients need information. People should know the names of the drugs they are taking, how to take them, how soon they can expect benefit, what the main side-effects are and how to minimise them, and what to do if there are difficulties they can't cope with. Some of this information may be given during the consultation, but it may not be retained. Written sheets or leaflets can be used to reinforce and expand on what has been said.

Increasingly, drug companies are including patient information in product packs, but this may not be available where drugs prescribed by their generic name are dispensed in bottles. A sheet covering the above points could be produced in the practice quite cheaply. The Defeat Depression Campaign leaflets 'Depression' and 'Depression in the Elderly' have sections on antidepressant treatment. The *Complete Guide to Psychiatric Drugs* (Lacey 1991), available from MIND, is intended for the general public and might be a useful addition to a practice library.

(c) Support

Many authors (for example Wilkinson 1989, Livingston 1990, Wright 1993,) consider that treatment by prescription alone is inadequate. Frequent short appointments mean that quantities of drugs can be kept small minimising the risk of suicide, and the opportunity to express feelings can be provided.

Regular longer sessions with a practice nurse – perhaps interspersed in the early days by telephone contact – may enable social difficulties to be identified and dealt with as well as support to be offered. A pilot study has demonstrated the feasibility of practice nurse support being provided for patients on antidepressant therapy (Wilkinson *et al.* 1993). Ordinary general-trained practice nurses received appropriate training for this task. One of the nurses involved in the study commented that learning about depression had altered her approach to all her patients. She was now very much more aware of the psychological aspects of health and illness.

To prevent relapse, treatment with antidepressants should continue for four to six months at the therapeutic dose. Longer courses may be necessary for patients who have recurrent episodes of depression (Paykel & Priest 1992).

2. Selective serotonin reuptake inhibitors (SSRIs)

These drugs are also known as 5HT-reuptake inhibitors. Examples are Sertraline (Lustral), Fluoxetine (Prozac) and Paroxetine (Seroxat). They are chemically unrelated to the tricyclics. They are often said to have fewer side-effects than the latter and to be much less toxic in overdose. This lower toxicity has led some doctors to consider that SSRIs might be more suited to general practice use.

The Effective Health Care review suggest that SSRIs are no more effective than older drugs. Side-effects are not necessarily fewer, merely different and they are also more expensive. Their use as a first-line treatment for depression would considerably increase NHS prescribing costs without significant benefit.

Research into these drugs continues, and their use is becoming more widespread. Recent opinion suggests that side-effects **are** less troublesome and compliance with treatment may be better. If this proves to be the case, treatment may be more effective, outweighing the increased cost. They remain controversial.

3. Monoamine-oxidase inhibitors

These drugs, for example isocarboxazid (Marplan) and phenelzine (Nardil), are sometimes used for patients who do not respond to tricyclic antidepressants. They are most often used by specialists because of potentially serious side-effects, especially a severe rise in blood pressure. They can interact with other drugs, notably over-the-counter cold preparations. There may also be dangerous reactions with some foods such as meat extracts, chicken livers, wines and some cheeses. Close supervision is essential for patients taking these drugs (Wright 1993).

Compound antidepressants, which consist of a tricyclic and either a minor tranquilliser or an antipsychotic, are not generally recommended because the doses of the individual drugs should be tailored to the patient's requirements.

Lithium is mainly reserved for the treatment and prophylaxis of bipolar disorder (manic depression). Patients require careful monitoring.

Figure 4.2 which summarises the salient points in antidepressant follow-up could be used as a basis for a written practice protocol.

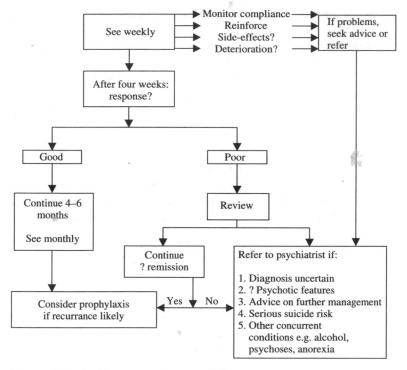

Figure 4.2 *Antidepressant therapy follow-up*

Social

As early as 1982 Mann and Jenkins pointed to the influence of social factors in predicting outcome for patients with depression in general practice. In their study it was the quality of the social networks, and relationships within the family that were the most important. An attempt to improve social support for people with depression seems, therefore, to be justified. It is important to identify the type(s) of support which might be beneficial.

Brown (1992) defines effective support as:

1. The presence of a close confidant.
2. Active, on-going emotional support from that confidant.
3. The avoidance, by the confidant, of making negative comments about the person needing the support.

This illustrates why counselling may be of particular value to people who have been bereaved, especially those who have been widowed. The counsellor becomes the replacement confidant, allowing the bereaved person time to rebuild his/her social network. Counselling can thus be seen as a social as well as a psychological intervention.

A further insight into effective forms of social support is given by Barbee (1990). Her research looked at the ways in which a helper provided support to a distressed friend. She noted four types of behaviour, two of which worked, and two of which didn't. This has lessons for professional helpers.

Positive behaviour included:

(a) Problem-solving – asking about stressful events and circumstances and making suggestions about how to cope.
(b) Emotional support – giving encouragement, affirming the person's ability, being sympathetic (which means accepting the person's feelings as valid).

Behaviours which were not helpful were:

(a) Belittling the problem – telling the person that their problem was not important or substituting one's own problems. Some nurses do this, mistakenly believing they are empathising ('I know how you feel – I've had that too').
(b) Avoiding the issue by pursuing their own agenda, changing the subject or concentrating on something else like reading the patient's notes while they are talking.

Problem-solving seems to be the most practical element of social support which can be given within the general practice setting. There are four parts to this:

1. Identifying problems
   Problems which are causing difficulties for the patient need to be recognised. The social and emotional factors associated with depressive illness are dealt with in more detail in Chapter 7.

2. Setting goals
   Realism is useful here. Patients need help to identify the things they **can** change. Steps should be small and achievable, goals appropriate to the situation. They must be agreed in dialogue with the patient, not imposed or ordered. 'If I were you' is generally an unhelpful phrase.

3. Providing information
   Help will often come from outside the practice team. In general help with finance, benefits and housing will be available from local authority or statutory agency. Help with difficulties relating to social

networks, for example, befriending, social skills training or support groups will come from the voluntary sector and help with work-related difficulties may be found from trade union or occupational health sources. It is useful if one person in the practice can take responsibility for compiling and keeping up to date a register of local sources of help. As a basic minimum, each practice should know how to contact:

- An agency offering bereavement support, for example local CRUSE branch.
- RELATE branch for couples counselling
- Group providing support for carers
- A general counselling service (in the absence of a practice counsellor)
- Citizens' Advice Bureau
- DSS office
- Samaritans
- Interpreting Service – if the practice population includes patients from ethnic minorities who do not speak English.

Details of locally agreed referral procedures for social services should be available, and be part of the induction process for new members of staff, including new partners and/or trainees. Referral difficulties often occur where the procedures are not followed.

The practice health visitor and district nurse's telephone numbers should also be easily to hand.

4. Encouragement

A positive attitude is important – 'you can change things' rather than 'poor you, isn't it awful'. By consulting the doctor or nurse, the patient has asked for help, not to have distress reinforced.

Achievement must be celebrated. This is a small, but vital step in the process of raising self-esteem. It is useful and may be motivating to offer a follow-up appointment. This is then used to praise success and, if necessary, take goal-setting another small step forward.

PHYSICAL

Depression in the presence of physical illness should be treated in the same way as depression without physical illness. Depression is common in people with chronic, painful, disabling or life-threatening illness. All the above aspects of treatment should be considered.

It can seem perfectly natural that a person with a long-standing illness might become depressed from time to time. The treatment of physical

57

illness is usually regarded as the priority in general practice, but the patient whose depression is recognised and treated may be able to cope more effectively with his/her physical condition, even terminal illness, and quality of life will certainly be better (Grieves 1993).

Community nurses, and specialist nurses working with terminally ill people often feel that referral to supportive services, such as MacMillan nurses or a hospice should come earlier rather than later in the illness. Patients and their families may cope more successfully with their condition if they know to whom they can turn should a crisis arise.

Alderman (1993) has described an innovative counselling support service set up by Elsye Hulse, a Macmillan nurse, which aimed to provide immediate help for outpatients who had just received a cancer diagnosis. The main value of the scheme was thought to be that patients knew there was someone to whom they could turn. Someone cared.

Practice nurses will meet patients with depression in their chronic disease management clinics. The focus of these clinics is, as their name suggests, to manage chronic disease – usually hypertension, diabetes or asthma. Most nurses have protocols or guidelines which they follow, but few of these allow for an assessment of mental state.

A worsening in coping skills may alert the nurse to the possibility of depressive symptoms. A more systematic approach might be to include a short mental state assessment in the clinic protocol, perhaps by using a screening questionnaire, or simply asking each patient how they feel in themselves.

People who seem to be depressed can be referred to the GP for further investigation. The nurse might also realise that a patient may wish to discuss problems which would take more time than the clinic setting allows.

In one practice, a group of nurses has dealt with this by offering such patients a further 10-minute appointment on another occasion, say the next day. This second appointment is used for problem-solving as described above. Should more help be required, the patient is then referred to the practice counsellor. This approach avoids disrupting subsequent appointments in a busy clinic, allows for the clinic aims to be met (particularly important where income generating targets are involved) and encourages the recognition of patient need.

SELF-HELP

Helping patients to help themselves is an important part of the care of people who are depressed. This emphatically does not mean telling people to 'pull themselves together'. In depression, that is exactly what people are unable to do.

General health advice is important, such as getting enough exercise, learning to cope with sleep problems and eating a healthy diet. Learning to relax is also useful, especially if anxiety symptoms are a feature of the depression, or if the patient feels under stress (Chapter 5).

The Defeat Depression Campaign's leaflet on Depression contains a useful section on 'How to help yourself'. There is also a chapter on self-help in *Depression: Recognition and Treatment in General Practice* (Wilkinson 1989), parts of which may be copied and given to patients.

CHAPTER FIVE

Anxiety and related problems

INTRODUCTION

Like depression, anxiety is a normal experience. When we encounter stressful situations such as an examination, a difficult task at work, a personal or family crisis, any one of us may feel anxious or tense. Such feelings may included headaches, finding it hard to relax, having difficulty with concentration, being irritable and sometimes snapping at family or colleagues with scant cause. More or less extreme outbursts of emotion such as anger or inappropriate laughter are commonly understood as due to 'stress'. There may also be physical symptoms like dry mouth, sweating, palpitations as heart rate increases, and shallow, rapid breathing.

These feelings reflect physiologically-useful mechanisms which release energy and prepare the body for action to counter danger (a stressor). This is known as the fight or flight response. Athletes use it positively when they 'psych themselves up' for a race. If physical action follows, the feelings disappear. The energy is used.

In modern life, 'fight or flight' may not be appropriate responses to particular stressors. But if the energy created is not dissipated in some way, tensions build up, and we say that the person is 'under stress'.

Anxiety and stress may be seen as synonymous, but whereas anxiety is usually considered negative, stress may have benefits. Not all stress is harmful. Some stress seems to be necessary for optimum functioning. It can provide motivation and it can lead to worthwhile change. Whether a stressor is perceived by an individual as a threat or a challenge may depend on a number of variables including personality type, the feelings of the person about the situation or event and his/her ability to cope with it (Sutherland & Cooper 1990).

ANXIETY AS ILLNESS

Anxiety becomes a clinical problem when it is too severe for the individual to handle, arises with no apparent trigger or occurs frequently in situations which would not normally appear threatening (Wilkinson 1992a).

About a quarter of patients in general practice have significant anxiety symptoms, but although anxiety may be obvious, it may not be the most important problem. About 70% of depressed people also have anxiety. Because the two conditions co-exist so commonly, depression is often misdiagnosed as anxiety (Casey 1993). It is depression which is the primary illness, and it should be treated accordingly. Wilkinson (1992a) suggests that trying to distinguish the two at general practice level is unhelpful from a treatment point of view.

What seems to be important is to distinguish 'trait' anxiety, which describes the habitually anxious personality, from a clinical anxiety state which requires some form of treatment. While acknowledging the existence of anxious personalities, there are dangers in dismissing frequent attenders at the practice as being in this category. Such people may be perceived as a nuisance and overly demanding (the familiar 'heartsink' patient). Receptionists, doctors and nurses collude to get them out of the surgery as quickly as possible. But this may mean that they never receive a proper assessment of their health care needs. An underlying depressive illness may be easily missed.

TYPES OF ANXIETY

While the most common form of clinical anxiety is the mixed anxiety/depression illness already mentioned, a number of specific conditions are also described:

- *Generalised anxiety* is excessive and unreasonable worry about life circumstances and social problems. It has usually persisted for 6 months or more. Symptoms include tension, irritability, concentration difficulties, and autonomic arousal characterised by such feelings as dry mouth, tremor, sweating, restlessness, hyperventilation and so on.

- *Phobias* involve irrational fear of objects, people or situations. Such fears are common. Many people have longstanding phobias, particularly of animals which arise in childhood. Whilst they may avoid the object of the fear, spiders for instance, no other disturbance of social functioning is present. Such phobias rarely present to the doctor and require no medical treatment.

  There are some phobias which are severely disabling. Agoraphobia is the best known. As well as fear of open spaces, there may also be fear of crowds and/or of leaving home. Commonly feared

61

situations include being in shopping centres, supermarket check-out queues and using public transport.

About two-thirds of agoraphobia patients are female. Symptoms usually start between the ages of 15 and 35. The condition often seems to have been triggered by a major life event. Patients may be afraid that something will happen to them in a particular situation – dizziness, falling, losing control of bladder or bowel, or of dying. The condition may have been started by a panic attack. Some sufferers become completely housebound and totally dependent on their spouse, other family member or friend for everything which involves going out. Agoraphobia may persist for years.

Social phobias, such as fear of answering the telephone or of eating in public places may be just as distressing, particularly for the person whose livelihood depends on meeting others. These fears, usually of doing something in a social situation which may prove embarrassing or humiliating, often arise in the teenage years.

Concurrent depression is common in both these types of phobia.

- *Panic attacks* are the sudden onset of severe anxiety which causes intense terror for the patient, often with feelings of impending doom. The associated physical symptoms – dizziness, palpitations, nausea, breathlessness and numbness in hands and feet – often lead people to believe they are seriously ill and may have a heart attack or stroke. These symptoms may be the result of accompanying hyperventilation (France & Robson 1986). In any event, panic attacks are extremely distressing for the sufferer, and if not adequately treated at an early stage may become severely restricting and lead to agoraphobia.

- *Obsessive-compulsive neurosis* is not common though obsessional symptoms may be present in depression. Sufferers may have a compulsion to carry out certain rituals to relieve anxiety feelings, for example washing hands to get rid of contamination. Alternatively there may be compulsive ruminations on a particular idea or the need to dwell on specific thoughts. The recurrent compulsions may become severely disruptive to the person's daily life and can cause considerable distress. The illness may become chronic.

- *Post-traumatic stress disorder* is a relatively recent term used to describe a reaction to a severely psychologically distressing event. It is usually said that the event should be outside the normal range of human experience. Depression is often a feature, as may be panic attacks and flashbacks (including nightmares) of the event.

Other terms which are sometimes used in relation to anxiety include 'free-floating' which means that symptoms may occur unrelated to obvious stimuli. The feelings may be present much of the time.

'Situational anxiety' refers to feelings which occur in particular anxiety-inducing circumstances. The person comes to recognise the circumstance, increasing apprehension and therefore the anxiety which ensues. Panic attacks may occur. (Wilkinson 1992a, Casey 1993).

RECOGNITION OF ANXIETY

Anxiety is an important feature of a number of other psychiatric disorders. Its presence as part of a mixed disorder with depression has been noted. It also occurs in such conditions as schizophrenia, dementias, in alcohol and/or drug abuse and in benzodiazepine dependence.

Physical disorder may need to be considered, in particular hyperthyroidism, hypoglycaemia and some cardiovascular, respiratory and neurological conditions. Some prescribed drugs such as corticosteroids, thyroxine and bronchodilators may cause anxiety symptoms. Excessive consumption of caffeine may be a factor (Wilkinson 1992a).

Though it may not be strictly necessary to distinguish between anxiety and depression for the purposes of treatment, there are a number of published scales to help the process. The anxiety and depression scale of Goldberg et al. (1988) is one such. In consists of two sets of nine questions, but it is so designed that the full set need be asked only if there are positive answers to the first four. The Hospital Anxiety and Depression (HAD) scale is also being increasingly used in primary care settings (Wilkinson & Barczak 1988).

Scales and screening instruments do not remove the need for a full clinical assessment. Their value, Goldberg and colleagues suggest, lies in the fact that they provide doctors with a tried and tested repertoire of questions, rather than the haphazard and unsystematic approach often used by non-psychiatrists.

A simple method which could be used by nurses in a variety of situations is to ask a short series of direct questions about the major symptoms of anxiety:

1. Have you been worrying a lot?

A positive answer should lead on to:

2. Do you feel keyed up and on edge?
3. Have you been feeling irritable?

4. Have you had headaches/dizziness/trembling/sweating/diarrhoea and at what frequency?
5. Does anything in particular bring on these feelings?
6. Are you worried about your health?

Possible sleep disturbance information should also be sought:

1. Do you have difficulty getting off to sleep?
2. Do you wake up frequently in the night?
3. Do you wake up early in the morning?
4. Are you sleeping too much?

It is also important to know how long the symptoms have been present. Answers to some of these questions may be suggestive of depression, for example early morning waking. Further assessment would be indicated.

Use of these questions could provide the nurse with a rational framework for making decisions about when to refer to the GP. The answers would provide a list of symptoms with which to make referrals credible.

THERAPEUTIC OPTIONS

Treatment begins with recognition and acknowledgement including explanations of the causes of anxiety symptoms. Patients often fear they have serious physical illness. It will be necessary to listen to the patient's beliefs about the illness, and to counter any erroneous or inaccurate ones.

It is important to distinguish beliefs about health which are wrong and damaging, from those which are culturally different. This can present enormous problems for primary care workers who have patients/clients from widely diverse ethnic backgrounds. Nevertheless, some understanding of the patient's view of his/her problems, and expectations of treatment, must be sought if care is to be acceptable and effective (Mares *et al.* 1985). Properly trained health interpreters should be used where necessary. The still widespread practice of using English-speaking children to interpret for their parents (often mothers) is both demeaning to women, and can result in misleading information being received by both patient and professional.

Treatment has psychological, pharmacological, social and self-help aspects. However, drug therapy is necessary only in severe illness for patients whose ability to function at home and at work is substantially impaired (Wilkinson, 1992a). Even in panic attacks, which usually occur suddenly and unexpectedly, a more measured approach is recommended than the immediate administration of a benzodiazepine (France & Robson 1986).

Psychological

These are probably the treatments of choice for most types of anxiety. They may be considered under three headings: counselling, relaxation training and behaviour therapy.

Counselling

This has been extensively discussed in the previous chapter. It may be of value for anxious patients where there is an obvious trigger such as relationship difficulties or bereavement.

Counselling is the major approach to treatment for people with post-traumatic stress disorder. It is sometimes offered by specialists following major disasters. Medication is considered to have little part in helping these people (Casey 1993). Counselling may be required both for disaster victims themselves and for workers from the emergency services involved.

Relaxation training

Relaxation is an integral part of many interventions designed to help people deal with feelings of tension and anxiety. It can be a useful treatment in its own right. The most commonly taught methods are based on learning how to alternately contract and relax groups of muscles in a systematic way, coupled with learning to recognise the feelings associated with each state. This may be combined with learning how to control breathing. Yet further methods rely on the visualisation of a pleasant place or event, perhaps under the direction of a therapist, a technique known as guided fantasy.

Training in controlled breathing may be particularly valuable for people who suffer from panic attacks. France and Robson (1986) believe that hyperventilation is an important component of panic and contributes to some of the symptoms because it reduces the amount of carbon dioxide in the blood. Slow, controlled breathing is, they say, incompatible with hyperventilation. Patients taught this skill can then learn to use it to moderate their feelings of panic.

Teaching relaxation skills to patients is not difficult. Nelson-Jones (1991) gives detailed instructions in his book *Practical Counselling and Helping Skills* (Cassell). A simpler version is given in *Anxiety: Recognition and Treatment in General Practice* (Wilkinson 1992a, Radcliffe Medical Press) which could be copied as a handout for patients. An instruction sheet for patients who experience panic attacks is given in France and Robson's book, *Behaviour Therapy in Primary Care.*

Teaching and learning relaxation does take time and commitment. The use of printed handouts and audiotapes, a variety of which are available, can considerably reduce the contact time between nurse or doctor and patient. Pace (1992) has described the inclusion of cassette tapes on relaxation in a practice library set up for patients. She suggests that tapes are particularly well-suited to teaching this topic because listening itself encourages relaxation.

Behaviour therapy

Behaviour therapy, which derives largely from learning theory, is employed to help patients substitute responses to situations and feelings which are more effective than their previous inappropriate or maladaptive ways of reacting. The aim is to help the patient learn a new response to an anxiety-producing stimulus. Change is always implied.

Relaxation training can be seen as a form of behaviour therapy. The term also includes cognitive therapy, which was described in the previous chapter. Here, the use of behavioural methods in the treatment of phobias, obsessional-compulsive disorders and other anxiety-related conditions will be described.

Primary care workers are probably most familiar with behaviour therapy from the treatment of agoraphobia. Techniques used include exposing the patient to the feared situation in a controlled manner. Exposure may be rapid ('flooding') or gradual ('graded exposure' or 'desensitisation').

The former method involves the therapist accompanying the patient into the feared situation and remaining there until the patient's symptoms subside. With practice, the patient learns to control the anxiety even in the absence of the therapist. This method of treatment normally requires a trained professional counsellor or psychologist.

Graded exposure works on the principle that every task can be broken down into small steps. A hierarchy of goals is set in which each goal contributes towards finally confronting the most feared situation. A system of rewards can be built in, and as each goal is achieved, self-esteem improves. A relative or friend may be enrolled as co-therapist. This method is suitable for use at home, but it takes time and commitment from the patient, family and therapist to avoid the programme running out of steam.

These and similar techniques can be used to treat other phobias and obsessive-compulsive rituals.

In theory at least, it might be possible for a suitably trained primary care nurse or doctor to undertake such treatment. In practice, it may be difficult to obtain the necessary training, and devote the time required in a busy practice. Most of these patients are therefore likely to be referred for psychological help.

This can present problems. Clinical psychology services may not be widely available, or easily accessible in every area, though a recent *Drugs and Therapeutics Bulletin* (1991) suggested that there were more of them than was commonly believed by many GPs. The bulletin also said that GPs are often unaware that they can refer direct to psychologists without going through the consultant psychiatrist.

Information about psychology and other services may not be easy to obtain. An interesting observation about this was made by a researcher looking into the accessibility of information for carers of patients with Alzheimer's Disease. She found that existing services rarely produced or disseminated information about themselves. There were two possible reasons for this phenomenon: either they had been there so long that they assumed everyone knew about them, or they were worried that if they did 'advertise' themselves, they would be overwhelmed with demands they could not meet. This applied to services in both the statutory and voluntary sectors (Gavilan 1992, Westminster Carers Association Survey, personal communication).

The first attitude, complacency, leads to GPs using inappropriate routes for referring patients, and then complaining that they cannot get the help they require when they want it. The second, fear, can lead to underuse of expensive services, and even withdrawal of funding because no need has been demonstrated.

Waiting lists for psychological treatment can be long – weeks or even months. GPs find this unacceptable, though closer enquiry will often reveal that many appointments are not kept. Patients who are flexible can often be seen at short notice. Many psychology services will offer assessments very quickly, though patients may have to wait for subsequent treatment.

Alternative sources of therapy may come from community psychiatric nurses, perhaps through community mental health teams which may operate independently of other psychology services. These teams often take direct referrals from general practice or even self-referrals by patients.

The voluntary sector may also provide support and treatment. Local MIND groups may be one such source. There is sometimes a reluctance on the part of GPs to refer patients to the voluntary sector – 'How do I know I can trust these people with my vulnerable patients?' Apart from the paternalism inherent in this attitude – adult patients are normally quite capable of making their own decisions – ignorance, both of the kind of organisations available locally and of the services they provide is the major factor in this reluctance.

Members of voluntary organisations often express the desire to work more closely with GP practices in their area. A policy of occasionally inviting such workers into practice meetings to explain the services they are offering could help to build confidence and improve communication.

Therapy in groups

Under the Health Promotion Clinic arrangements introduced with the 1990 GP contract, groups of all kinds proliferated in general practice settings. Among these were stress and anxiety management groups/clinics. Now that newer health promotion banding arrangements are in force, many of these groups probably no longer exist, but some may be useful.

Running stress management groups is within the capabilities of nurses with experience as group leaders – health visitors for example. However, these groups probably should be seen as protective rather than therapeutic in clinical terms. They will be considered later.

Anxiety management groups require a higher level of skill (for example Childs-Clarke *et al.* 1989, Casey 1993) and should be run by appropriately trained professionals such as community psychiatric nurses, psychologists, members of community mental health teams or counsellors. They may offer such interventions as relaxation training, cognitive-behavioural therapy and social skills and assertiveness training.

Groups can be a cost effective way of providing support and treatment in health centres, where there is sufficient space. One therapist can treat a number of patients at the same time and patients can offer support to each other. It is often helpful for people to know that their problems are not unique. Group methods could probably be more widely used.

Social aspects

Much anxiety is related to social circumstances and difficulties. Emotional and relationship problems are particularly relevant. Among elderly people worries about being unable to cope at home may be significant. Some studies have indicated the value of GP practice-attached social workers for helping these people. For example, Rushton and Briscoe (1981) describe a study which looked at the kind of work attached social workers did, and concluded that clients benefited from the multidisciplinary approach. This way of working is still far from the norm although authors continue to point to the advantages (for example Burke 1992, Ruddy 1992).

Traditional 'casework' seems to be the favoured method of intervention. Rushton and Briscoe define this as psychological help given with the aim of improving social functioning and modifying attitudes and behaviour. It was this kind of work which was found to be most useful by a social work team which set up a Stress Management Clinic in the Paddington area of London (Wolf 1992, personal communication).

Social workers are also likely to have knowledge of, and access to a wide variety of local services and organisations. Yet a social worker based for one session a week in a small health centre in an area of high deprivation, reported herself underused. The main reason appeared to be poor communication with other professionals in the health centre in which there was no tradition of team working.

Problem-solving techniques are probably one of the most effective ways of helping that can be used by GPs or nurses in primary care (Chapter 4).

Self-help

There are three aspects to self-help in this context:

1. Attention to general health, to taking adequate exercise, eating a healthy diet and all the usual healthy lifestyle advice.
2. A simple approach to discovering personal ways of coping with anxiety symptoms. This might include noticing what kind of actions tend to reduce anxiety symptoms, and to keep doing them. In this respect, alcohol and drugs would be inappropriate. Tobacco is also a dangerous prop – but trying to give up smoking while suffering anxiety symptoms is probably taking on too much.
3. It is sensible to avoid doing anything which makes the symptoms worse – provided that this does not interfere with a planned treatment regime.

Practice nurses and GPs will need to be aware of any of their patients who may be undergoing behavioural therapy with another professional in order to avoid advising anything which could undermine the treatment. An example might be the patient who finds the therapy hard going, and who asks his/her doctor for medication instead. This kind of situation underlines the need for good communications between professionals to minimise the danger of manipulation.

Patients can be encouraged to think for themselves of strategies which might help and to carry them out. A selection of leaflets, books and audiotapes could be kept in a practice library to facilitate this process. Suggestions and sources for this material will be found in the Resources section.

Pharmacological

Thinking about the place of drugs in the treatment of anxiety disorders has been extensively revised in recent years following the increase in knowledge about tranquilliser dependency.

The most commonly used drugs for anxiety are the benzodiazepines, of which diazepam (valium) and lorazepam (ativan) are probably the best known. Temazepam is widely used as a hypnotic.

All of this group of drugs are effective anxiolytics and sedatives. The choice of drug is said to be based more on commercial than any other criteria, the perceived differences being due more to pharmaceutical companies' need to sell more drugs than to differences in the drugs themselves (Lader 1989). The risk of dependence, which may occur after very few weeks' use, has led to a considerable decline in new prescriptions. There remain large numbers of long-term users.

Most authorities consider that their use should be reserved for short-term treatment of severe disabling anxiety and insomnia. Wilkinson (1992a) cites studies which have shown that benzodiazepines may be no more effective than a range of straightforward psychological techniques in over half the patients for whom they might be considered. In a study which compared anxiolytic treatment with brief counselling and support by the GP, the latter was just as effective as the former, and took no more GP time in over 60% of patients. Other patients may do better with a combination of drugs and psychological support.

In the mixed anxiety/depression illnesses common in general practice, antidepressants are the drugs of choice. Many antidepressants also have a significant anxiolytic effect.

Alternative drugs for anxiety include beta-blockers – which alleviate some of the physical symptoms – and a newer preparation, buspirone (Buspar). This drug has been launched with claims that there is no risk of dependence, claims which experience suggests should be treated with scepticism. Like the antidepressants, it has a delay in onset of action, making it unsuitable for short-term anxiety, and its use is still considered problematic (Casey 1993).

A normal anxiety response to a stressful situation, for instance an examination, should not be treated with medication. Doing so may impair performance. Training in relaxation techniques may be more appropriate.

Some recent authors (for example Mead 1992, King 1993) suggest that the anti-benzodiazepine movement may have gone too far, and that these drugs still have a place in general practice.

Withdrawing from tranquillisers

Encouraging long-term users of these drugs to reduce or abandon their dependence is generally considered to be good practice. While this may be the case, it is important that the views of patients should be taken into account when advocating withdrawal.

The average GP list is said to contain about 50 long-term benzo-diazepine users. King and colleagues (1990) have pointed out that these patients are a diverse group which does not necessarily conform to the media-stereotype of middle-aged women with personality difficulties. Patients are not passive receptacles for pills. Many may believe they have a continuing need for the drug, and many people seem to manage their use in positive ways.

None the less studies suggest that about half of long-term users would like to withdraw. The Mental Health Foundation has recently published a booklet which provides guidelines for both the prevention and treat-ment of benzodiazepine dependence (Russell & Lader 1993). The authors suggest that simple techniques, even a letter from the GP to all long-term users, could result in at least 20% of them giving up, or sub-stantially reducing their intake. For others, a programme of withdrawal should be planned and implemented, with on-going support. In all cases, withdrawal should be gradual. Sudden stopping of the drugs can lead to severe, sometimes life-threatening consequences.

People withdrawing from tranquillisers will always need support. While only about a third may suffer withdrawal symptoms, Tovet (1992) has suggested that the process of change which has to be gone through while withdrawing will always be painful. She believes that there is no alternative to meeting and learning to deal with this pain if healing is to take place, and withdrawal is to be successful and permanent.

Many people will need greater support than their GP or practice nurse will be able to provide, and alternative sources will have to be sought.

Such help may be available from community mental health teams, or from voluntary organisations like local MIND groups. National MIND publishes a nationwide directory of help for tranquilliser users (Murray *et al.* 1991). Groups may not be easily accessible in all areas, or may be part of more general drug and alcohol misuse services. Tovet (1992) has described a service set up in Camden for tranquilliser users which could provide guidelines for others wanting to set up similar projects.

Sleep disturbances

Problems with sleep are commonly associated with depression and anxiety. People may experience difficulty getting to sleep, may wake frequently during the night, or may wake early and be unable to get back to sleep. Some depressed patients may sleep too much.

Self-help measures are well known. Some of the more usual ones which may be advised are:

1. Have a regular routine – go to bed at the same time every night.
2. Avoid sleeping during the day.
3. Do not eat a large meal just before going to bed.
4. Have a warm, milky drink at bed-time, but avoid tea, coffee, alcohol and other stimulants.
5. Cut down on caffeine (tea, coffee) intake during the day.
6. Do not read or listen to the radio in bed unless you find it especially relaxing. In particular, avoid thrillers.
7. Do not lie in bed worrying about sleep. If you can't get to sleep in about half an hour, get up and do something else until you feel tired.

King (1993) suggests that the use of benzodiazepine hypnotics may not be unreasonable where self-help measures fail, provided there is no underlying psychological disturbance. Others (for example France & Robson 1986) believe that drugs may cause more problems than they solve.

Self-help measures may appear to fail because they are often unsystematically and inconsistently applied. People often believe that they sleep less than they actually do.

The child who doesn't sleep can cause extreme distress to the parents. In general, the GP or practice nurse will not be the most appropriate person to help these families. They should be referred to the health visitor without delay. He/she is likely to have the most up-to-date knowledge and experience of this problem. In particularly intractable instances, it should be for the health visitor to refer on, usually to a clinical psychologist, unless the GP has expertise in behavioural techniques.

If parents are at the end of their tether, then drugs may be considered for short-term relief, but they may be ill-advised. Their effects are unpredictable, they often don't work and they are difficult to stop.

Sleep diaries may be a useful way of recording what is actually happening, both for adults and children. Information to be recorded includes:

- time of going to bed;
- time of getting to sleep;
- number of times of waking during the night;
- any action taken;
- time of getting back to sleep;
- time of waking in the morning.

Adults might also like to record how they feel in the morning, whether alert or tired. This may provide some surprises for the adult who believes he/she 'doesn't sleep a wink all night'. Some anxiety may be relieved.

For the parents of a non-sleeping child, patterns of behaviour may be revealed which, if modified, may improve the child's sleeping habits and relieve the parents' anxiety.

CHAPTER SIX

Schizophrenia in primary care

Not long ago a young black man attended his GP surgery for his regular injection of an anti-psychotic drug. When this patient arrived, the GP had already begun her morning surgery. The procedure was that patients arrived, booked in at reception and had to wait their turn as there was no appointment system. Most arrived early in an attempt to beat the queues which inevitably built up as this was a popular GP. The result was that our patient had to wait for more than an hour. He was well known to the receptionists as likely to become noisy and even violent if he had to wait long. This indeed happened and by the time his turn came he was already causing some anxiety to others in the waiting room. The system was simply too inflexible to accommodate the needs of this young man. The practice had no nurse.

Another GP complained that a discharged psychotic patient was so ill-prepared for his move into the community that he regularly panicked at night and called out his GP, much as he would have called his nurse in hospital. After enduring this situation for a week in which he was called out every night, the exhausted doctor not surprisingly arranged for the patient to be readmitted.

The bizarre, anti-social and often noisy behaviour of some mentally ill people can be disturbing in general practice settings. It may not only alarm other patients in the waiting room, but also disrupt the work of staff who are inadequately trained to cope. Actual numbers of patients involved may be small – about seven per GP on average (Jenkins 1992b) – but the problems caused can be way out of proportion, so much so that in many practices the objective of everyone is to get rid of the patient from the premises as quickly as possible.

Many patients who have serious mental illness prefer to be treated in the relative normality of their GP surgery. In principle this is fine, but:

1. The GP, though willing, may not have the facilities nor the support to offer the kind of comprehensive medical and social care many of these patients require. Some GPs have even suggested that they may

be more willing, and better able to offer improved care for people with depression and anxiety if they could be confident of good back-up support for their psychotic patients.

2. Patients may fail to keep their hospital outpatient appointments. To the hospital they may be 'lost to follow-up'. To the GP they have lost their specialist back-up. Communication between the two, GP and hospital, may be too poor to allow the situation to be easily resolved, when all that is required may be a phone call.

3. In practice, anti-psychotic injections may be delegated to a practice nurse, who will probably not have a mental health nursing qualification. She may have only hazy knowledge of the nature of the drugs used and of their side effects, and she may be unaware even of the name of the patient's key worker.

4. A further problem relates to the physical health of these patients. The *Health of the Nation* (1992) has pointed out that mentally ill people have extremely high death rates from common physical illnesses like heart disease and cancers. Yet mentally ill people are often excluded from health promotion activities in general practice perhaps because they are perceived as a nuisance by the receptionist who is responsible for booking clinic appointments – 'You won't get any sense out of her, she's mad!' The high prevalence of smoking among mentally ill in-patients is obvious to any health-aware visitor to a psychiatric unit. In the rest of the hospital, smoking will probably be banned, or at least confined to designated areas. The feeling that psychiatric patients cannot benefit from the general health advice available to the rest of the population seems neither fair nor logical. If there is to be a real improvement in the general health of mentally ill people, ways will have to be found of making health promotion initiatives accessible to them in spite of the very real difficulties.

Better understanding of the nature of serious, long-term mental illness and of the needs of patients would mean better care and, perhaps, less disruptive behaviour which often seems to be caused by frustration.

SCHIZOPHRENIA

Schizophrenia is the commonest of the serious mental illnesses, often known as psychoses. While the clinical aspects of these diseases (signs, symptoms and medical treatment) may vary, the principles of quality care will be common to all.

The psychoses are primarily disorders of thought, in contrast to depression and anxiety which are disorders of mood or affect. Psychotic illnesses are said to be characterised by lack of insight, detachment from reality and bizarre symptoms such as delusions and hallucinations (Tredgold & Wolff 1984). The distinction between neurotic and psychotic forms of psychiatric illness is now thought to be less useful. Depending on the severity of their illness, patients may show features of both types.

Modern systems of classification of psychiatric illness, such as the American Psychiatric Association's DSM III, rely on defining groups of symptoms which are then used to determine diagnosis (Casey 1993).

There has been a huge amount of criticism over the last few decades about the diagnosis of schizophrenia. Many psychiatrists believe that it is not a single disease, rather a group of related conditions. Some consider that the term should be abandoned (Hill 1993), others that it is useful because it signifies that the sufferer has a serious condition whose effects should not be trivialised (Murray, 1993).

Young, black males are more frequently diagnosed as schizophrenic than any other group, and are over-represented among those compulsorily detained under the *Mental Health Act*. Most black people assume that this is due to inherent racism in the psychiatric services and the police and believe that psychiatry is used as a form of social control (Fernando 1993). Listening to black people discussing their experiences of this can be challenging for a white health professional. There is real and understandable anger.

Whatever the truth about racism in psychiatry, the incidence of schizophrenia when narrowly defined (so-called 'first rank' schizophrenia) is fairly constant across cultures at about 1 in 100 people (Leff 1992).

Symptoms of schizophrenia

Symptoms are often divided into positive and negative. Most patients present with acute positive symptoms which include:

- *Delusions* – firmly held false beliefs, often bizarre. People may believe that thoughts are being inserted into, or removed from their heads by outside forces such as electricity, radio or witchcraft. Care must be taken in interpreting delusions, since there is obvious scope for cultural misunderstandings. In particular some firmly held religious beliefs may be wrongly attributed to delusions.
- *Hallucinations* – defined as perceptions in the absence of stimuli; that is seeing, hearing or even tasting things which are not there. Most commonly, people with schizophrenia 'hear voices'. These may

be very disturbing, commanding the sufferer to damage themselves or others. 'They speak to me in order to deceive and derange and force me into . . . paranoia . . . ' (Bayley 1993).

- *Thought disorder* – may be apparent in muddled speech where thoughts do not appear to follow a logical sequence. *Inappropriate affect* where mood does not seem to match expressed feelings may also be present. Other conditions such as drug misuse, temporal lobe epilepsy and organic brain lesions need to be excluded as possible causes of these symptoms.

Negative symptoms include poverty of speech, social withdrawal, loss of initiative and drive, and blunt or flat mood. These symptoms are often chronic and may be due to either schizophrenia itself or concurrent depression which is common.

Onset is commonly in late adolescence or early adulthood, somewhat earlier in men than in women. It is rare in childhood, but may occur for the first time in later life (Lawrie 1993).

Causes

The causes of schizophrenia are still unknown. Research has looked at genetic, biological and psychosocial aspects. Newton (1988) considers that a genetic component is now firmly established, though others have disputed the evidence. Leff (1992) states that siblings of a schizophrenic patient have a nine times higher risk of developing the disease over the general population. For the children of a schizophrenic patient the risk is 12 times higher, rising to 40 times for the children of two schizophrenic parents.

Abnormalities in brain anatomy and physiology have been investigated, as has the association of later schizophrenia with virus infections *in utero* and possible birth injury, but there are no clear conclusions.

Intensive studies of environmental, psychological and social factors are likewise inconclusive. Abnormalities of communication style have been observed in families with a schizophrenic member. These abnormalities include over-protective and more intrusive mothering, more marital disharmony and inconsistent, vague use of language. It is difficult to decide whether these so-called abnormalities pre-date the illness or are caused by it (Newton 1988).

Onset of schizophrenia is often preceded by a clustering of life events. These are more likely to be precipitating factors than actual causes.

77

Outcome

In Britain about a quarter of patients recover completely from a first episode and do not have another for at least five years. Some patients remain free of symptoms for many years and live relatively normal lives in the community. As Leff (1992) comments, this is a much better outcome than most hospital based practitioners – who commonly see patients who do least well – would expect.

A major WHO study, quoted by Leff, has shown that in some Third World countries outcome is even better than this. Nearly half of patients recover and do not relapse for several years. The reasons are not fully understood, but may be related to more accepting and tolerant family care than is usual in the West.

Treatment

This is divided into two main areas:

1. drug treatment for acute, positive ('florid') symptoms which are the usual presenting features and which dominate relapse;
2. psychosocial measures designed to deal with negative, chronic symptoms, rehabilitate sufferers, support carers and prevent relapse.

Drugs

Neuroleptics, also known as antipsychotics or major tranquillisers, are used. There are several distinct chemical groups, meaning that different drugs may suit different patients. Trials of treatment may be necessary to find the drug of choice.

Dosage also varies considerably from patient to patient. Side-effects can be serious, therefore dosage needs to be kept at the lowest level possible consistent with symptomatic control. Acute symptoms are normally dealt with initially using chlorpromazine (largactil) or haloperidol (haldol, serenace). Patients may be treated in hospital during this phase, particularly if the presenting symptoms include aggressive or highly disturbed behaviour. A calm, undemanding hospital regime may be beneficial. Once symptom control is achieved, medication will be adjusted to individual requirements.

Drugs commonly used in maintenance therapy include those mentioned above, and others such as fluphenazine (Moditon, Modecate) and flupenthixol (Fluanxol, Depixol). Clozapine (Clozaril) is a newer preparation claimed to be effective in patients whose symptoms have been resistant to other drugs. However, it may cause serious neutropenia and patients therefore require regular monitoring including white cell counts.

Drugs may be given orally or by injection as depot preparations. Oral medication causes fewer side-effects but compliance in patients with poor insight is a serious problem. Monthly depot injections may be preferable. The frequent professional contact which the latter regime requires has benefits in the increased opportunity for assessments of symptom level and social care needs. Unfortunately, this may also be the point at which care breaks down, if the injection is given by an insufficiently skilled and aware person.

Side-effects

Atropine-like effects such as dry mouth, blurred vision, constipation and sedation may be troublesome with some of the lower potency neuroleptics.

More serious are neurological effects:

- dystonia and dyskinesia – parkinsonian-type involuntary movements, usually of the mouth and throat, or disturances of posture;
- akathisia – physical and mental restlessness and agitation ('restless legs');
- akinesia – lack of movement.

Delayed effects ('tardive dyskinesia') are potentially very serious and may be irreversible.

There are a variety of methods used to overcome these effects, but the main principles of treatment are:

1. use the lowest dose of antipsychotic possible, consistent with symptom control and the prevention of relapse;
2. do not continue any drug used for side-effect relief longer than is absolutely necessary (Crammer & Heine 1991, Tantam 1992, Mortimer 1993).

Psychosocial care

The *Health of the Nation* target A is 'to improve significantly the health and social functioning of mentally ill people'. Even though outcome measurements will not be available before 1994/5 and the targets may be refined towards the middle of the decade, there is already plenty of anecdotal evidence suggesting much room for improvement.

It was apparent early in the KCW study that practice nurses were anxious about giving depot injections to schizophrenic patients. GPs were concerned about increasing numbers of these patients on their lists (at least twice as many as Department of Health figures suggest). These anxieties were not confined to inner London. Discussions revealed a widespread perception that community care arrangements were underfunded and would fail. It would be the GP who would have to pick up the pieces. Psychiatric services were described more than once as 'not user friendly'.

Some of these problems are acknowledged in the *Mental Illness Key Area Handbook* (Department of Health 1993):

> 'Mental Illness has remained a poor relation in NHS . . . management priorities. Services . . . have been fragmented and poorly coordinated . . . poor information . . . inappropriately targeted resources . . . alliances not developed to their full potential.' (pp. 12–13) and 'use of mental health services is . . . a reflection of historic circumstance . . . (rather) than a reflection of need.' (p. 34)

Primary prevention of schizophrenia is not yet a viable option. Secondary prevention definitely is. Long-term, carefully monitored treatment with neuroleptic drugs controls positive symptoms and prevents relapse, though often at the expense of damaging side-effects. However these drugs do not influence outcome in social terms. Many patients with good symptomatic control still show considerable social disability. Negative ('deficit') symptoms are not helped by drugs (Shepherd 1992).

Tantam (1992) suggests that a systematic approach to the social care of patients with schizophrenia is helpful. His model has four elements:

1. *Stress monitoring.* People with schizophrenia have more difficulty than others in dealing with stressful situations. They may react by withdrawing inappropriately or exhibiting erratic behaviour so it may be best to avoid this kind of situation altogether, if it can be anticipated.
2. *Stress management.* It is neither possible nor desirable to avoid all stress, therefore patients need to learn how to manage everyday stresses in an acceptable way.
3. *Coping strategies.* People need to learn how to face unavoidable, demanding situations such as a job interview.
4. *Social skills training.* This helps to make patients more independent and more assertive.

These four elements can also be applied to the support required of carers since there is evidence that the attitudes of carers influence outcome. In particular those patients whose relatives show what is known as high expressed emotion ('EE') seem to do less well. Relatives under excess stress are likely to show high EE, that is they may be over-critical, hostile or too involved with the patient. Patients seem to do best in a calm environment which makes few demands on them (Leff 1992, Shepherd 1992).

Practice nurses and GPs may not be actively involved in this kind of care, but in so far as they have these patients and their families on their lists, they are in an excellent position to monitor care, and to alert the care manager or key worker if arrangements appear to be breaking down.

The care programme approach

This approach to care for the long-term mentally ill came into effect in April 1991. It was designed to create a network for care in the community for all patients about to be discharged from a psychiatric hospital, and all new patients referred to specialist psychiatric services. It was not confined to those patients with well-recognised social needs who would be referred to a social services care manager.

All patients in the categories above should have an individually written plan agreed with the patient and his/her carers, informal (relative or friend) and professional, and a named key worker. The key worker would normally be a mental health professional, usually a community psychiatric nurse (CPN) or social worker. The plan should be regularly reviewed.

For patients discharged to GP care from specialist services (not just hospital psychiatrists) adequate information about the care plan must be provided for the GP, with the patient's agreement. Clinical responsibility needs to be clear, particularly for prescriptions and for physical health care (Key Area Handbook, Department of Health 1993).

Practice nurses should question whether they are wholly competent to give anti-psychotic medication. In a recent survey which examined practice nurses' roles in mental health, Thomas and Corney (1993) found that whereas 89% of nurses said they dealt with mental health problems, 87% felt inadequately trained.

Turner (1993) quotes a number of authors who suggest that CPNs who give these injections may have reduced their other interactions with patients. Since this appears undesirable, some CPNs have reacted by referring patients to GPs for their medication, leaving themselves free to deal with other nursing issues. It is by no means clear that such extra interventions actually happen, and CPNs may be depriving themselves of useful opportunities for patient contact. There are also implications for continuity of care.

Though these findings may be of prime importance to CPNs, they are also matters of which practice nurses should be aware. Practice nurses who regularly give depot injections should consider the following:

1. Do they fully understand the nature of the drugs they are giving, and the potential side-effects?
2. Is there clear guidance available, preferably in the form of a practice protocol, for the actions which should be taken if adverse effects occur?
3. Are they aware of the name of the key worker for all such patients, and is regular contact maintained?
4. Do all patients' carers have adequate support?

Practice nurses who feel they need more training for this role should take steps to obtain it preferably through their FHSA nurse adviser or facilitator. The UKCC *Code of Professional Conduct* (1992) places a duty on nurses to admit limitations in knowledge and to decline tasks which they are unable to perform in a 'safe and skilled manner'. Practice nurses sometimes feel that their jobs could be at risk, or relationships with their GP employers may suffer, if they become more assertive about their training needs. Sadly, if they fail to acknowledge limitations, it is their whole career which could suffer. Some GPs may need reminding that nurses are personally accountable for their professional actions, and can lose their registration if they do not behave responsibly.

If any existing patient does not appear to have a key worker, or has no contact with specialist services, it may be advisable to consider referring him/her for review and further assessment, but always with the patient's consent.

An earlier survey by Thomas and Corney (1992) showed that links between GP practices and mental health professionals vary considerably, with some practices having many links and others few or none at all. The authors question the equity of this state of affairs, but also acknowledge that the quality of the links is as important as their number.

Shared care, which has become widely accepted in maternity services and for people with diabetes and asthma, also seems to have potential for the care of mentally ill people. A GP, a psychiatrist and a CPN in south London described such a scheme, which proved acceptable to patients. A patient-held record card was felt to be a useful aid to communication both between patient and professional, and between professionals. At least one patient commented that it helped him explain to police that the drugs he was taking had indeed been prescribed by his doctor.

The patients involved in the pilot scheme were all suffering from schizophrenia or other chronic mental illness. Compliance was described by the authors as 'surprisingly good'. The concept of a patient-held shared record card was said to improve patient autonomy.

The main barrier to further development of this scheme was staff attitudes. Psychiatrists were apparently unhappy about patients having access to records (which was not mandatory at the time) and believed that local GPs were either not able, or did not want to participate in care for this group. Community nurse managers showed little interest. GPs were the most positive but 'patients' enthusiasm far exceed that of psychiatrists, general practitioners, nurses or managers' (Essex *et al.* 1990).

These issues have assumed greater importance since April 1993, when GP fundholders were enabled to purchase mental health services for their patients. There is an opportunity to ensure that services purchased from specialist providers, for example psychiatrists and CPNs, are used to benefit those whose need for specialist care is greatest. The danger may be that these highly trained but relatively scarce professionals could be diverted to providing care for people who are depressed and anxious, which from the GP's perspective is a much more substantial group. Such a move would be disastrous for those with long-term, chronic mental illness.

'Sectioning'

This term is often used when mentally ill people are compulsorily admitted to hospital. Such admissions are allowed in England and Wales under the *Mental Health Act* 1983. The circumstances governing them are clearly defined. The Act covers people who are 'mentally disordered' through:

- mental illness;
- mental impairment;
- severe mental impairment;
- psychopathic disorder (a persistant disorder which leads to abnormally aggressive or irresponsible conduct).

Promiscuity, other immoral conduct, sexual deviancy and drug/alcohol dependency are not criteria for admission under the Act. Some professionals consider that this creates confusion, especially where drug and/or alcohol abuse exacerbates a psychotic illness.

People may be admitted for:

- assessment (Section 2);
- treatment (Section 3);
- emergency admission (Section 4);
- guardianship (Section 7).

Admissions can only be made if the patient would otherwise require voluntary admission, or if his/her own health or safety, or the safety of others is at risk. Applications for admission under Section 2 must be made by the patient's nearest relative or an approved social worker to the hospital managers and two registered doctors. The admission may last for up to 28 days.

Guardianship

The rules of guardianship provide the means whereby a person may be enabled to live in the community in as normal a way as possible, but as a safeguard be required to live in a designated place and be required to maintain contact with the appointed, named, 'guardian'. The person can be returned to hospital if the terms are not adhered to.

Some provisions may vary under the Acts for Scotland and Northern Ireland. Further details about the Act are available in a fact sheet from the Royal College of Psychiatrists from which the above information is taken.

The physical health of the mentally ill

That people with serious long-term mental health problems also suffer disproportionately from serious physical illness like heart disease and cancers has already been mentioned. Not only do GPs miss depression, but psychiatrists frequently miss physical illness (Jenkins 1992a). While there are undoubtedly clinical issues here, the problem has been given extra emphasis in the *Health of the Nation*. Improving the health and social functioning of those with serious mental illness does not just mean improving their mental health. Yet the physical health of these people seems to have received much less attention.

In the audits conducted for the KCW study a number of patients with schizophrenia who were also insulin-dependent diabetics came to light. These patients were extremely high consumers of practice time, with consultation rates three or four times the average and though no detailed assessment was made, their care seemed to be chaotic and unplanned. A more systematic approach might have been beneficial to both patients and practice.

The multiaxial approach to assessment advocated by Jenkins is said to provide GPs with a more comprehensive method of diagnosis and management which addresses all the patient's needs. This kind of approach could also be used by nurses to assess nursing and health care needs.

CHAPTER SEVEN

Prevention of mental illness

Activities aimed at preventing illness have been going on in primary care for years. Among the earliest were probably immunisation. Since the early 1980s, prevention of heart disease and cancers has become prominent, with a great deal of effort going into helping people change unhealthy aspects of their lifestyle – to give up smoking, cut down on saturated fat and take more exercise. These activities are encouraged in general practice by financial incentives.

Until relatively recently though, the only primary care professionals specifically trained in prevention were health visitors. When health visiting started in the nineteenth century with the Voluntary Visiting Association in Manchester, the major concern was with reducing the appalling infant mortality due to squalor, lack of hygiene and ignorance amongst parents (CETHV 1977). In later years the focus shifted to child development and the early detection of problems such as hearing impairment which if untreated may lead to language delay and learning difficulties. The health visitor is often perceived by others in primary care as working only with the under fives because of this historical concern with the health and welfare of children, but children do not exist in a vacuum. They have mothers and families. Probably the most valuable aspect of health visiting is that which takes the mother as its starting point, supports her and helps her learn to be an effective parent in both practical and psychological terms. Lack of care in childhood has been shown to be a cause of adult depression (Newton 1988).

Among all the existing primary care interventions aimed at preventing illness, the support of parents is almost the only one which has any potential for preventing *mental* illness.

DEFINITIONS

Preventive activity is commonly divided into primary, secondary and tertiary (Jenkins 1992c):

- *Primary prevention* implies that a disease is prevented from happening at all. It means either identifying the cause and countering it as in immunisation, or identifying the risk factors and taking steps to reduce or modify them. An example of the latter would be the man with a raised blood cholesterol level who is advised to change his diet in order to lower the level, and therefore reduce his risk of having a heart attack.

  Bereavement is a known risk factor for depression. Offering the bereaved person support at the time of the loss may enable the process of mourning to be gone through in a healthy way, preventing the development of a clinical depression and removing the need for drug therapy.

- *Secondary prevention* measures shorten the length of an illness, reducing the period during which the individual suffers distress. They also lessen the likelihood of long-term adverse consequences. For instance, the early detection of precancerous states by screening reduces the need for mutilating surgery for cervical cancer and, research suggests, can reduce the death rate (*Health of the Nation* 1992). Early detection and prompt treatment of hypertension reduces the risk of a stroke.

  The potential benefits to mental health of early detection of depression have already been noted (Chapter 3).

- *Tertiary prevention* is concerned with limiting the disability caused by chronic illness or injury. It enables people to make the most of residual abilities and prevents pre-existing conditions getting worse. Severely injured people may, with good social care and appropriate modifications to their homes, be enabled to live as near a normal life as possible.

  Careful monitoring of drug regimes in schizophrenia will prevent relapse and minimise side effects (Chapter 6).

Newton (1992a) has offered a definition of prevention which seems to overlap the concepts of primary and secondary, or to combine elements of primary prevention and early detection. She suggests that prevention is 'action intended to reduce the incidence of mental illness amongst people who are relatively free of . . . symptoms or who are suffering from . . . symptoms not severe enough to be defined as cases (i.e. not diagnosed)'. This definition is said to avoid the danger of labelling as 'ill' those who are experiencing normal reactions to stressful situations. Work with people who have a small number of symptoms can be considered prevention rather than treatment.

Primary prevention of schizophrenia has been seen to be unrealistic in the present state of knowledge. In terms of depression and suicide, however, the situation is more promising.

THE POTENTIAL FOR PREVENTION

In her extensive review of the literature, Newton (1988) identifies two major approaches to prevention:

(a) the disease (or medical) model;
(b) the health (or health promotion) model.

The disease model involves identifying those individuals who are at high risk of developing a disorder and targeting preventive measures at them. The health model targets the general population with measures known to be preventive of disorder for a few and assumed to be health promoting for the rest.

It is the latter approach which has been used to address the problem of heart disease. Newton quotes the principle stated by Rose in 1981 that 'a large number of people exposed to low risk . . . (will) produce more cases than a small number . . . exposed to high risk.' This principle has been used to justify mass population strategies for reducing heart attack deaths. The premise is that if everyone takes action to lower their risk a little, this will have more effect on death rates than if the relatively small number of high risk individuals is targeted.

This principle may also apply to mental illness to some extent. But depression differs from heart disease in an important respect. In heart disease, most deaths occur in low to moderate risk groups, whereas with depression most cases are found in high risk groups. For example, a bereavement is much more likely to trigger a depressive illness in women with poor social networks and low self-esteem than in women with a good sense of self-worth, and supportive relationships. Newton suggests that our knowledge about depression is at a stage where we can identify high risk groups with some confidence.

A further reason for concentrating here on a disease or 'medical' model of prevention is that general practice, and much of primary care, is a medical setting. Disease-based approaches are therefore likely to appear to have the most relevance, and to be more acceptable to workers. The best chances of success appear to lie with measures targeted at those at highest risk.

PREVENTION IN PRACTICE

Suicide

Two of the three targets for the mental illness key area in the *Health of the Nation* set a standard for the reduction of suicide rates; one for the overall rate, and one for suicide in the seriously mentally ill.

In 1991 there were 5567 deaths from suicide (and undetermined injury) in England. This is 1% of all deaths annually and is greater than the number of deaths from road accidents. The suicide rate in young men aged 15 to 24 has risen by 75% since 1982. Suicide is the second most common cause of death in males aged 15 to 34. Rates of suicide are twice as high in men as in women. Suicide also accounts for 8% of all working days lost through death.

It is possible that suicide figures are artificially low. Suicide was a criminal offence within living memory and considerable stigma still attaches to the idea. Of those who kill themselves:

- 90% have some form of mental disorder usually depression;
- 40% have consulted their GP in the previous week;
- 33% have expressed clear suicidal intent;
- 25% are psychiatric outpatients.

(Source: Department of Health 1993)

Risk factors

Certain groups are known to be particularly at risk, especially if also suffering from depression. About 15% of people with depression will eventually kill themselves (Wilkinson 1989). Psychiatric patients, especially those with schizophrenia or affective psychoses are at greatly increased risk. 1 in 10 will kill themselves. Alcoholism and drug abuse compound the risk.

In general, risk increases with age. Older men are more likely than younger people to kill themselves especially in the presence of other risk factors such as bereavement. The reasons for the recent increase in suicide rates in young men are unclear. High rates of male unemployment, and AIDS have been suggested, but evidence is inconclusive.

The menopause may increase the risk for women who can become depressed when children leave home. Young women with children, though at risk of depression, are less likely to take their own life. An increase in suicide among Asian women has recently been highlighted. A facilitator colleague, herself Asian, believes that this may, at least in part, be due to non-recognition of depression among this group.

The English word 'depression' has no exact translation in languages from the Indian sub-continent, but this does not mean that Asian women do not experience depressive illness. They just describe it differently.

Severe physical disability or life-threatening illness can increase the risk both of depression and suicide. Mutilating surgery, especially for cancer, is an important factor as is any condition which predisposes to social isolation, such as chronic disability causing people to become housebound, or communication difficulties like deafness and visual impairment.

Other chronic social difficulties such as housing or financial pressures; marital or relationship problems; unemployment, sudden redundancy or worries at work are all possible precursors of depression and suicide, especially where there are multiple problems. Socially isolated people with severe communication problems, especially those who have difficulty making and sustaining interpersonal relationships are likely to be at high risk.

A personal or family history of previous suicide attempts is also important since about 10% of those who try but fail will eventually succeed in killing themselves, many within the following year. For this reason it is unsafe to regard all attempts (parasuicide or deliberate self-harm) as attention-seeking gestures (Russell & Hersov 1983).

The choice of method is important in assessing the degree of risk. The more violent the method chosen, the more likely it is to succeed. Car exhaust fumes account for 33% of male suicides, drug overdose for 66% of female suicides, the drug most commonly used being paracetamol.

In a recent review of the evidence on suicidal behaviour, Williams & Pollock (1993) concluded that in addition to social factors there were some psychological factors which increased vulnerability. These are difficulties in regulating emotional responses – often characterised by hostile and demanding personal relationships; hopelessness about the future; and poor interpersonal problem-solving skills.

Unfortunately there is as yet no way of predicting which patients in primary care will try to kill themselves. The most promising preventive measure seems to be improving the detection and management of depression (Effective Health Care 1993). It has been suggested, too, that primary care teams should participate in local audit of suicides and undetermined deaths, especially of people with mental illness who have been in contact with mental health services (*Health of the Nation*: 'First Steps' 1992). This is now happening in some areas.

Suicide may not seem a major problem for the individual practice team. In a practice with about 6000 patients there is likely to be only one suicide a year. This means though, that in the area covered by a DHA or purchasing consortium with a population of about 500 000 there may be 50–60 suicides a year. The number of parasuicide cases may be 10 times higher, which represents a significant workload for local accident and emergency units. Measures to improve the aftercare of the latter group would involve much closer liaison between A&E units and GP practices in their area. Evans (1993) suggests that an act of deliberate self-harm may provide a 'window of opportunity' for positive intervention. The patient is likely to be particularly vulnerable following the attempt and may be receptive to sensitive offers of help. By no means all hospitals have detailed arrangements for the assessment and follow up of these patients by specialist teams, although this has been recommended since 1984. GP fundholders may be in a position to influence hospital trusts to provide such services.

Depression

The second of the aims of the KCW study was for the facilitator to help practices devise ways of identifying and offering support to people at risk of becoming depressed (Chapter 2). A number of ways in which this might be achieved were considered. No method is without difficulty, and all have implications for practice workload. One possibility was keeping a register of 'at risk' groups among the practice population, for example the bereaved, carers and so on, but manual registers are time-consuming to compile, and of little use unless they are regularly updated. They would also need to lead to some kind of action – a visiting service for the vulnerable perhaps. However, in the absence of a method of identifying those people who are in most need of support, this would be an unprofitable task.

Computers can of course be used to identify members of 'at risk' groups if appropriate software is available – which is by no means always the case. Again, targeting the most vulnerable could be a problem since there may be no way of knowing from patient records who those people are. The limited nature of the information in GP records and the difficulties of reading them are well-known to anyone who has used them to conduct audits. Computers may make information easier to retrieve, but they do not necessarily improve its quality. The KCW study was also under a further constraint at the beginning, in that some of the intervention practices did not have computers.

A way of assessing health risk already exists in many practices, in the new patient health checks, and the well-person checks that many practice nurses offer. The majority of these checks use protocols designed to identify people at risk of heart disease and cancers (for example Fullard *et al.* 1987). They are almost always devoted to assessing physical health. 'Stress' might be acknowledged as a cardio-vascular risk factor, but it is rarely quantified – questions about it might be confined to 'Are you under stress?' Yes or no. For the project it was decided to use this existing framework and to add a mental health component to the assessment. The aim was to design a method which would:

90

1. Enable practice nurses to assess the mental health risk status of patients during a normal health check or well-person clinic.
2. Identify those at higher risk.
3. Provide a means by which the GP could be alerted to high risk patients.
4. Provide guidance to practice nurses on the kind of support that might be realistically offered, bearing in mind the time pressures that all in general practice are under.

The method was eventually piloted by a nurse in one of the central London intervention practices, and by a number of other practice nurses in various parts of the country. All the nurses involved were ordinary practice nurses with no specialist mental health training. They all had close support from their local primary care facilitators, the latter being an essential element in giving them the confidence to take part in the pilot (Armstrong 1993a).

ASSESSING RISK

A semi-structured nursing interview was used to identify risk factors, which were then recorded on a health risk card (Figure 7.1). The card was designed to fit into the Lloyd George style GP envelopes that all the research practices used. This meant that space was limited. Only brief headings could appear on the card, and there was little space in which to write details.

The interview was designed to be part of a general health check. Since it concentrates on social and relationship difficulties it might also be adaptable for use as an assessment of social needs for people who are already depressed (Chapter 4). Nurses were advised as follows:

1. To complete the physical part of the health check first. This was so that the patient would be relatively relaxed, and some measure of understanding should have been established between nurse and patient.
2. To obtain agreement from the patient before the social part of the check began. It was to be made clear to people that answering questions about personal matters was entirely voluntary. In practice very few people refused. Many expressed appreciation of the chance they were given to discuss their problems. Nurses felt that asking the questions added to their care an extra dimension which had been missing before.
3. The interview was not to be seen as a method of counselling.

1	2	3	4	5	6	7	8	9	10	11	12	13	14

RISK INDICATOR

NAME	DATE			
Bereavement Relationship	Yes	No	Male		Female	
Marital Problems Date of Divorce	Yes No		Living Alone		Yes	No
Single Parent No of dependent children Recent Childbirth	Yes No .... Yes No		Social Contacts: Supportive / Unsupportive			
Caring for Disabled Person Yes No Relationship .... Details Any support?			Recent change of residence Yes No (eg.new immigrant) Details:			
Physical Health: Any disabilities Sensory Physical			Employed / Unemployed How Long?			
Serious physical illness Details:			Difficulties at Work Details:		Yes	No
Family history	Yes	No	Financial Problems		Yes	No
Details: Medication:			Details:			
Family Problems	Yes	No	Housing Problems Details:		Yes	No

Figure 7.1   *Health risk assessment card*

4. It was not a method of diagnosing depression although it might raise suspicions in the nurse. Any patient who appeared to be already suffering from depression was to be referred to the GP.

5. The method looked only at risk factors. It did not attempt to assess vulnerability or coping skills, both of which might modify the degree of risk.

Guidelines about the risk factors were provided for nurses but they did not specify the questions in detail. Rather they explained how the risk factors might influence health. Nurses were free to frame the questions in whatever way seemed most appropriate.

The risk factors

Bereavement

Though this is a major factor, and one whose effects can be felt many years after the event, it should not be assumed that all bereaved people will suffer from a depressive illness which requires treatment. Parkes (1986) suggests that those bereaved patients whose depression symptoms could be described as pathological were those in whom the grief reaction was either prolonged, delayed or both.

Support offered to a newly bereaved person by the primary care team, GP, practice nurse or district nurse, if offered at the time of bereavement, may be preventive. But Newton (1988) suggests that even this type of support is likely to be most effective if targeted at people who have few alternative sources of help.

The most serious loss is likely to be that of a spouse or partner, followed by parent, sibling or child. Abortion and stillbirth are bereavement too. Just as important for some people could be the loss of a friend if particularly close, or indeed a pet for a person who has few human contacts. The loss of a homosexual partner may be especially distressing for the one who is left; gay people may have few family ties, and therefore little support.

Marital and relationship problems

Divorce or separation from a partner, either heterosexual or homosexual, may or may not be a risk factor. The partner who has found a new relationship may be at less risk than the mother abandoned with several young children. Separation from a violent partner may actually be a relief. Therefore it isn't enough to know that a separation has happened. Equally significant is the way the person feels about it, and whether there are still conflicts. Problems might include disputes over the custody of children, loss of the family home and financial difficulties. Divorce is a significant cause of female poverty (Corob 1987).

Difficulties in existing relationships may also become apparent, including violence and other forms of abuse and, commonly, psychosexual problems.

An interesting observation often made, is that employed, single women with no dependants are at less risk of depression than married women. The reverse seems to be true for men for whom marriage is said to be protective.

At the design stage of the assessment it was anticipated that psychosexual problems were something which nurses might find difficult to handle. They were advised to avoid long discussions about areas in which they had little expertise. It was sufficient to recognise and acknowledge the existence of a problem. The second part of the assessment made suggestions about finding suitable help for patients. In practice, nurses reported few difficulties in setting boundaries and in knowing their own limitations.

Parents and children

Mothers with three or more dependent children, no confiding relationship and no job outside the home have already been seen to be at increased risk of depression (Chapter 3). Single mothers with a variety of social difficulties and little support are therefore an important high risk group.

Postnatal depression is three times as common as depression in the general population, and not just in single mothers. Most new mothers should be in touch with a health visitor, who may use the Edinburgh Postnatal Depression Scale (EPDS) as a screening tool (Cox *et al.* 1987). A patient who is new to the area and just registered with the practice may need help to contact the health visitor.

It should be automatic for practice nurses (and GPs) encountering mothers with young children who are in difficulties to refer to the practice health visitor. The health visitor will have knowledge of, and access to, all appropriate local sources of support for this group.

Long-term caring

A spouse or adult son or daughter caring for an elderly person with dementia, a parent with a disabled child, or a relative caring for a mentally ill person may be at high risk of becoming depressed themselves. It is all too easy for general practice staff to focus on the needs of the sick person, and neglect the carer. For example, elderly carers often complain that they are refused home visits by practice staff because they are seen as relatively fit. But it may be impossible for the wife of a man with dementia to leave him behind. If she is to get to surgery, she will have to take him with her. This may be a major undertaking if she has no help, and she may therefore give up the attempt, sacrificing her own needs when a more flexible attitude to home visiting might have resolved this problem. Alternatively, local carers' groups may offer a 'sitting-in' service to allow the carer the opportunity to shop, visit the hairdresser or go to the doctor or optician.

Physical health

Physical and mental health are closely linked. It is worth remembering that people who are mentally ill have more physical illness than others (Jenkins & Shepherd 1983). However, there are two main aspects of physical illness which might increase the risk that the patient will also become depressed:.

1. Sensory deprivation (see under Social isolation).
2. Any condition that is disabling, painful or life-threatening. Imminent major surgery, for cancer for instance, may increase risk, especially for people who have little family support.

Psychiatric history

A previous family or personal history of mental illness is a risk factor for a subsequent episode but asking about this may be perceived as intrusive by the patient. The relevant section on the card was therefore designated 'Family History' to avoid the use of words like psychiatric or mental. It seems advisable to confine questions to something like 'Have you ever been depressed?' and 'Have you ever needed treatment for this?' Details could be sought later from medical records if necessary. It is important not to duck these questions, though.

Other family problems

A variety of other family difficulties may be associated with increased risk of depression. For parents, this might be related to an adolescent son or daughter with problems of moodiness, truant or drug misuse.

Adults who have been sexually abused as children may be at increased risk. Some nurses are reporting increasing numbers of people admitting to this previously hidden problem. Help for such people may not be available locally at present.

Social isolation

It is the quality of social networks that is important, not their size. Lonely people may have large numbers of casual acquaintances but few close friends in whom they can confide (Berg & Piner 1990). People who have difficulty making relationships may be helped by social skills training from a counsellor or psychologist.

Living alone does not of itself mean loneliness. Many people who live alone do so from choice. Nor should it be assumed that those who live alone will necessarily have many unmet health needs, but social isolation may be caused by physical disability, particularly sensory deprivation such as hearing or visual impairment. Help for these people, and for people who are physically disabled and housebound may be found through social services and, frequently, the voluntary sector.

Moving house

A change of residence, especially if this involves moving away from family and friends may be a source of distress for many people, above all for a mother with young children who has no job of her own. Older people may retire to a completely new area, cutting themselves off from previous sources of support such as work colleagues or relatives.

Immigrants may be at risk for all the above reasons but the plight of refugees deserves special mention. Many come from countries where civil war and repression are endemic. Most will have fled from torture; political, racial or religious persecution; unfair imprisonment; deliberate killings of relatives and associates and denial of the basic social freedoms we in this country take for granted (Source: Bulletin of RASU – Refugee Advisers' Support Group, May 1992).

Many who come to Britain will themselves have been detained or tortured. Many have also lost family members in horrific circumstances. The majority have little English when they arrive; they may have no money, inadequate clothing and nowhere to live. It would be surprising if they were not traumatised by their experiences. They do not understand the health and social security systems and many are dependent for help on voluntary organisations. Their first contact with the NHS might be when they try to register with a GP – and they encounter immediate suspicion from practice staff about their entitlement. Refugees and asylum seekers are entitled to free NHS treatment. They are not illegal immigrants. In order to properly assess and meet their needs, help may be needed from interpreters and/or specialist advisory groups.

96

Work-related problems

Unemployed people often become depressed especially where there are other problems such as poverty, but in the pilot study it was apparent that problems at work might be equally significant. Examples of such problems are fear of redundancy and racial or sexual harassment. Bullying in the workplace is considered by some to be a much underrated cause of a large amount of distress and anguish (Adams, 1992).

An appropriate trade union, or occupational health department may be useful sources of help for people in these situations, but external counselling and/or legal advice may be necessary.

Other factors

Long-term financial problems, debt and poverty, and housing problems are often sources of risk. It is unnecessary for the nurse to ask for details of income. This would be intrusive. But many people are unaware how debilitating chronic money worries can be, neither are they always aware of their benefit entitlements nor how to get help to resolve debt.

The type of housing in which the patient lives is not significant, provided it is appropriate for their needs. Many people do, though, have long-term problems with their accommodation which may relate to size and location, but might also involve state of repair, level of rent or mortgage repayments, overcrowding and even noisy and disruptive neighbours.

Practices in university towns may well be familiar with the problems students experience being away from home for the first time or during examinations. A recent spate of suicides among students has highlighted the fact that even young people who seem to have everything to live for may become depressed.

IDENTIFYING PEOPLE AT HIGH RISK

Once risk factors have been recorded people at higher risk can be identified. The cut-off point used was four or more factors. This was an arbitrary decision, but the pilot study showed it to be not unreasonable.

In inner London there was a large proportion of people in the high-risk category. To make the work manageable, the threshold was raised here to six or more factors. Overall the number of people assessed in inner London was small, and it is possible that already known high-risk individuals had been selected by the practice.

ALERTING THE GP

The 'Risk Indicator' across the top of the card was designed to alert GPs to high risk individuals at their next appointment. The number of risk factors identified was totalled and a corresponding number of boxes was highlighted.

OFFERING REALISTIC SUPPORT

Nurses using the assessment were advised to offer support only to those in the high risk group. They were advised to allow other people the possibility of returning for help if necessary. Help was not to be 'pre-scribed' nor were referrals to be made. A problem-solving approach was advocated, similar to that which was described in Chapter 4. This is a different kind of approach from the one commonly used by general nurses. The idea behind it is that helping people identify and solve their problems for themselves is likely to be more effective than either giving advice or taking over the decision making.

Advice is often ignored, however well-meant. Decision making by the professional rather than the patient saps self-esteem, reinforces feelings of inadequacy and creates dependency. The stages in a problem-solving approach might be:

1. Help the patient identify a problem which he/she would like help to solve.
2. Get the patient to list all possible solutions as creatively as they wish. This could be done between appointments as 'homework'.
3. Help the patient delete all solutions which are impracticable. What is left is, by definition, possible.
4. The patient should now decide which solution to go for, make a definite plan to carry it out, and set a time limit.
5. At this stage the nurse may need to provide information about suitable sources of help in the community, for example advice agencies, legal centres, social service departments, other health professionals, self-help groups and so on. Direct referrals should not be made. The patient must be allowed to choose which agency to use, or whether to use one at all. The nurse's role is confined to providing information which enables the choice to be an informed one. She must also continue to offer non-judgmental support to her patient, whatever choice is made and whether she agrees with it or not.
6. The patient should be offered a further appointment at which progress will be reviewed. Any success, however small, which the patient has had, should be celebrated in some way. Even a small

success, if achieved personally by the patient, will provide a boost to self-esteem, enhance the feeling of control that the patient has over his/her life and give encouragement to tackle further difficulties.

Throughout the process it is important that the nurse maintains an encouraging attitude, affirming the patient's ability to make changes. While accepting and acknowledging the reality of the patient's problems – in effect giving permission for the person to be distressed – it is vital to avoid colluding with the distress. In other words, to say 'I accept that this is causing you to be unhappy. Let's see if there are ways of making it better', rather than 'Poor you, isn't it awful' (see Brown 1992, Newton 1992b). The first is positive. The second reinforces the distress.

Some of the nurses in the pilot study reported that many patients needed only the opportunity to talk through their problems, with the nurse as a sympathetic listener. Nurses regarded this as good use of their time. They were not trained counsellors, and did not find it difficult to admit the limits of their skills or to provide information about professional counselling services if this was required.

In order to support the nurses in information-giving, a problem-oriented list of national and local helping agencies was provided by the facilitators. The list was so successful in the intervention practices of the KCW project and in the risk assessment pilot study referred to here, that many GPs also requested copies. It was later adapted into a problem-solving booklet for patients to be available in the practice waiting room.

A booklet like this could be fairly simply produced using desk-top publishing software, perhaps by health promotion units, facilitators or FHSAs. It would need to be fairly short, concentrating on major sources of help and advice, and, above all, it must be local.

CHAPTER EIGHT

Promoting mental health

WHAT IS MENTAL HEALTH?

Many doctors still find concepts of positive health, physical or mental, difficult to accept or understand. Health may be seen as simply an absence of symptoms of illness. Yet it can be argued that health and illness are not mutually exclusive (Sartorius 1992). Good nutrition and physical fitness are achievable even in the presence of serious medical problems. Most people would agree that those who enter sporting competitions for the disabled do enjoy a large measure of health.

Trent (1993) discusses the medical view of mental health in detail, but while pointing to the problems inherent in using the presence or absence of illness as a method of definition, he does not at this point present an alternative concept.

In an earlier piece (1991) he has suggested that five senses – trust, challenge, competence, accomplishment and humour – are central to being human. Decrease or loss of any one of these will affect the individual's ability to function normally. While this idea may throw some light on mental health, it is probably not enough on its own to provide a definition.

Dines and Cribb (1993) have reviewed the most frequently used definitions of health. The medical view is seen as too restricting. It neither allows for the evident health of the physically disabled as described above, nor does it take into account that, though free of symptoms of illness, a person may still be worried, anxious and lonely, and therefore not entirely healthy.

Conversely, the well-known WHO definition that health is a state of 'complete physical, mental and social well-being' is seen as too idealistic. Could anyone really be so healthy? In the view of many, another flaw in this view would be that it does not mention emotional or spiritual health.

In spite of the difficulties it is this second definition which is taken by many in health promotion as their starting point. The key concepts are that:

1. Health involves the whole person; body, mind and social relationships.
2. Health means well-being, feeling good about oneself, not simply being well or not being ill.

These ideas are perfectly respectable and accepted by health professionals when only the word 'health' is used. Add the word 'mental' and the whole perspective changes dramatically.

Asked to brainstorm 'mental health', a group of experienced general nurses on an advanced course came up with a list of psychiatric diagnoses. They could be forgiven. Mental health to many people is not simply, as Trent suggests, defined by mental illness, it is synonymous with mental illness. It doesn't help that psychiatric nurses and other specialists often refer to themselves as mental health workers, when clearly they are not.

A more helpful, and more practically useful view of mental health needs to acknowledge the 'health' dimensions of wholeness and well-being as well as the psychological implications of the word 'mental'. It also needs to encompass the concepts of 'coping'. A clinical psychologist suggested that mental health was having the ability to deal with all the vicissitudes of life without becoming ill (Armstrong 1993b).

WHAT IS MENTAL HEALTH PROMOTION?

Discussions about the nature of health promotion and its place within the NHS can become extremely wide-ranging and diffuse. They can seem to have little relevance to day-to-day work with patients and clients.

The term 'health promotion' itself has gained currency since the early 1980s. Before that health promotion units were known as health education departments and their main function was the supply of health-related literature for patients. As the cost of leaflets rose, less emphasis was placed on their distribution and new ways of raising awareness of health matters were sought, but as Dines and Cribb point out, the vagueness of the debate has made it sometimes very difficult to set boundaries and define responsibilities for those who work in the field.

Fascinating as the academic arguments might be, from a practical point of view boundaries are essential in order that effort is concentrated in areas which will bring the greatest benefit for the most reasonable cost (Tolley 1993). It is also necessary that activities are appropriate to the settings in which they take place. For instance, providing good quality housing at affordable prices may well be health enhancing (for mental as well as physical health), but it is not the business of the National Health Service (Newton 1992a).

The Concise Oxford Dictionary defines 'promote' variously as 'to help forward, to encourage, to support actively', and 'to publicise and sell'. In summary, then, promoting mental health may be seen as helping, encouraging, supporting and publicising measures which seek to enhance the psychological well-being of individuals and communities, and to improve their ability to cope with adverse circumstances. 'Coping' in this context has several aspects. It means changing what can be changed, accepting and learning to live with what can't, and recognising the difference.

Mental health promotion is an integral part of promoting health in general, not something to be practised only by specialists. For those who work in the NHS – and in the context of this book for those who work in primary care – it should be directed towards helping people cope with those areas of their lives over which which the NHS might be said to have some influence, notably illness and disease whether physical or psychological.

This is not to say that health workers should not concern themselves with the wider aspects of health. Who better to understand and explain how political and economic decisions affect the health of individuals, families and communities? The point is that health workers are faced with helping their clients cope, on a day-to-day basis, with actual and immediate concerns. Blaming 'them' (government or anyone else in authority) for the problems, however justified, serves only to deflect attention from things which can be changed. Even within the constraints of an unsympathetic political climate, there is much that people can do to help themselves.

It is unrealistic to think that GPs or practice nurses can attempt to fill the gaps for people whose social networks are inadequate. Nor is it the responsibility of most primary care workers to intervene directly in people's social circumstances or relationships, except in so far as these impinge on mental and physical health. Where such interventions may be warranted, for instance where marital problems appear to be at the root of a depressive illness or be placing individuals at risk, professionals can help people identify and mobilise the many sources of support which exist in every community (Jenkins 1992c).

THE SCOPE OF MENTAL HEALTH PROMOTION

Given that commonly used definitions of mental health and of health promotion all have disadvantages, it is possible to tease out some guidelines for primary health care workers, and to suggest some ways in which they might be supported by health promotion units.

Essential components of mental health promotion seem to be:

1. The prevention of mental illness.
2. The provision of mental health-aware services.
3. Mental health education.
4. Psychologically-aware support for staff.

Prevention was discussed in detail in the previous chapter. The social aspects of depression were highlighted as was the need for practices to have a detailed knowledge of local sources of help for their patients and clients.

The importance of such knowledge is difficult to overestimate, yet it is an area which typically receives scant attention. Practice nurses rarely have time allowed during their working hours to enable them to seek out the information. Health visitors and district nurses usually have local knowledge in abundance, but the value of it may be unrecognised by their colleagues.

Facilitators, whether employed by FHSAs or health promotion units, are well placed to set up, disseminate and maintain a local information database. Often themselves ex-health visitors, they are used to finding and making contacts with both statutory and voluntary agencies.

THE PROVISION OF MENTAL HEALTH AWARE SERVICES

Awareness is by no means as simple a matter as it may seem. It is obvious that treatment will affect the health of patients – that is its aim. But the environment in which care is delivered, and the attitudes of those delivering the service are also vital components. The practice which wants to promote the mental well-being of its patients must not only seek to detect illness, but should create an atmosphere which makes the experience of consulting a doctor or nurse as health enhancing as possible. There are a number of ways in which this might be done.

Practice organisation

General practice can sometimes be seen as operating in the interests of staff rather than patients. Receptionists, whose role in creating the atmosphere and ethos of the practice is vital, are frequently depicted as protectors of the doctor rather than as welcoming to the customer. Some practices even display drug-company produced posters which exhort the patient, in a variety of ways, not to waste the doctor's time. These seem more likely to create resentment than cooperation.

Petty rules such as those which state that one 10-minute appointment is for one person only may be understood by the practice to mean that if two people want to see the doctor together, they should make a double appointment. Patients may think that the doctor refuses to see more than one person at once. Where does this leave the husband and wife who want a joint discussion about something which effects them both? And how do you separate the needs of the child from those of the mother?

Practices could usefully ask themselves, and their patients, the following questions:

1. How accessible is our practice to mothers with young children, older people and those with physical disabilities?

Consulting rooms at the top of steep stairs, inadequate toilet provision, inflexible home visiting arrangements, inefficient appointment systems, and unwelcoming waiting rooms with too few seats may all cause unnecessary discomfort, anxiety and contribute to aggressive behaviour.

You may not be able to change the geography of your surgery overnight, but you can make sure elderly disabled people don't have to climb steep stairs, hold the ante-natal clinic on the ground floor and adjust your appointment system so that you don't have too many people waiting at one time.

2. How culturally aware are we? Do we know about the health beliefs of our main ethnic minority groups, and do we make sensitive and intelligent use of our local interpreting service?

A colleague tells a salutary tale of a non-English speaking Punjabi woman in some distress who was asked, through an interpreter, to describe her problem. The interpreter translated her words literally: 'My family is drinking my blood'. The unfortunate lady was compulsorily admitted to a psychiatric unit suffering from psychotic delusions. But the Punjabi words might have been more accurately conveyed in English by 'I cannot cope with all the demands my family are making of me', or 'They are draining me dry'. The reaction of the professional to this would have been very different (Dhillon, personal communication).

It is well worth remembering that English is not the only language which uses metaphor to describe feelings. Translation is not enough. Interpretation is also essential.

Coping with aggression

A feature of general practice in recent years seems to have been both an increase in demand by patients and an increase in aggressive behaviour. As a practice manager put it, 'Its not that people are any sicker, they just demand more'.

To some extent this increase in demand, especially for more responsive services concerned with social and psychological aspects of care (Coyle *et al.* 1993), may have been fuelled by political initiatives like the *Patient's Charter*, but consumerism as a general movement predates the Charter by many years. Consumerism in health care was inevitable and it can be a positive force for change.

Nevertheless, some GPs and their staff working in inner-city practices feel that aggressive behaviour from patients is becoming more common. For those who are faced with this problem, it may be worth seeking formal training in dealing with it. The FHSA, local health promotion unit or community mental health team may be able to help.

In some instances some form of protection for staff may be necessary, though this would inevitably reduce ease of access and may be undesirable. A balanced approach is necessary. When incidents occur, for example between patient and receptionist, the practice team should review and reflect on the incident in an atmosphere of calm which apportions no blame and allows all concerned to learn positively from what happened. The aim is to prevent recurrence.

Unfortunately a common reaction to severe aggression, especially violence, is to freeze. This is not helpful, but training may be required to break this pattern of behaviour. Braithwaite's book, *Violence: Understanding, Intervention and Prevention* provides some useful exercises (published by Radcliffe Professional Press, 1992).

Meeting psychological health needs

Whether this happens in a practice, or not, seems to be largely a matter of practice culture and is related to the way in which the GPs view the large numbers of people they see who are 'sickened and dis-eased but not clinically ill in a medical sense' (Marsh 1993). Marsh's solution is to employ a counsellor.

Although a counsellor provides an extra therapeutic option and a resource for the practice team in helping people who are distressed, experience suggests that the mere presence of such a person does not automatically improve the recognition and management of psychological and psychiatric disorders. Warner *et al.* (1993) offer some support for this assertion in their recently reported study of the effects of a community mental health service on the practice and attitudes of GPs. Though the team was considered helpful in dealing with patients with psychosocial problems, the authors believed that GPs themselves risked becoming de-skilled.

For benefit to accrue from a counsellor appointment, it seems essential that the counsellor is well integrated into a practice team. This means not only carrying a case load, but also supporting and educating other members. As Marsh suggests, this allows team members to develop an increased awareness of interpersonal and social issues that affect patients. The counsellor may also be able to help with relationship problems within the team.

Working as a team

Teamworking in primary care is considered by many authors to improve patient care and provide a greater sense of achievement for staff (Pritchard & Pritchard 1992). Lack of identifiable teams was one of the more important factors limiting the scope of the facilitator's interventions in the KCW study (Chapter 2). Not only was it extremely time consuming to inform practice members individually about stages in the project (where there are no regular team meetings there is often no reliable system of communication within the practice) but it was also impossible to involve practice teams in developing their own protocols. Yet the importance of good teamwork is nowhere more apparent than when considering mental health care. No one member of the team has all the answers. This book has considered many ways of improving the psychological aspects of patient care. Without teamworking, none of it will happen.

The Health Education Authority's Local Organising Teams (LOTs) provide a framework within which primary care teams can develop their effectiveness, and play their part in meeting the *Health of the Nation* targets. Primary care facilitators, health promotion units and/or FHSAs should be able to provide information about local activities. An alternative source is the HEA's Primary Health Care Unit in Oxford.

A team-based course on the Primary Care of Mental Health is also being developed under the auspices of the Royal Institute of Public Health and Hygiene. A distance learning pack for primary care teams based on this course will become available early in 1995.

Working with the secondary care services

It has been acknowledged elsewhere that to improve mental health care in general practice, the greatest need is to improve the skills of GPs, practice nurses and others who work in this setting. Most psychological disorder seen in general practice does not require referral to specialists, and since there are too few specialists to cope with the vast numbers of people in primary care who suffer from such disorders, were they to try, it is those extremely vulnerable people with psychotic illness who would miss out.

This does not mean that there is no primary care place for specialists, but rather than direct intervention with clients, they may be better used developing an educative and supportive role. In particular there seems to be considerable scope for improving cooperation and understanding between practice nurses, health visitors and district nurses on the one hand, and community psychiatric nurses on the other.

The *Health of the Nation* publication 'Targeting Practice' (1993) provides examples of a number of initiatives of multidisciplinary groups contributing to the care of people with mental health problems, but in few instances are there explicit examples of different professional groups of nurses coming together.

One area where working together could be beneficial is in the promotion of general health for those with long-term mental illness. The *Health of the Nation* (1992) points out that this group has higher death rates than the general population, not just from suicide but from heart disease and cancers as well.

Improving the health of mentally ill people does not just mean their mental health, but the author has had extreme difficulty in finding examples of general health promotion activities aimed at these people. MIND appeared not to have considered the issue at all. A request for help in the nursing press received no response.

Among the few positive ideas found was a scheme by a community dietitian and her colleagues in Durham to run 'Look After Your Heart/ Look After Yourself' courses, not for the mentally ill but for adults with severe learning difficulties (Howson 1991, unpublished). The scheme, which proved more successful when carers were also involved, was able to demonstrate some lifestyle change in participants.

Many practice nurses are experienced in a wide range of health promotion activities in primary care settings. There appears to be enormous potential for them to develop, alongside CPNs and health promotion specialists, ways of improving access to health in its widest sense for mentally ill people. Some ideas might be:

1. Improving stress-handling skills so that mentally ill people do not have to resort to alcohol or cigarettes; devising ways of helping mentally ill people give up smoking, if that is what they want.

2. Improving nutritional knowledge, not only about healthy eating *per se*, but also to enable mentally ill people in the community, many of whom live alone, to feed themselves healthily on a day-to-day basis. Community dietitians could also help with this.
3. Encouraging mentally ill people to increase their physical activity where possible, by improving access to sports and leisure facilities.

One such programme has involved a facilitator (who has a psychiatric nursing qualification) in the Midlands in cooperation with a local authority-run leisure centre. The centre provides a meeting place once a month for people with dementing illnesses and their carers. Care assistants provide a gentle exercise regime for the patients, while their relatives are free to make use of the centre in whatever way they wish. This is a healthy alliance in action. It provides mental, physical and social health-enhancing opportunities for elderly mentally ill people and those who care for them.

Sadly, this kind of scheme is often given low priority by health service managers. Funding may be precarious, and there may be little commitment to professional involvement. The facilitator above was allowed six months to set up his initiative and was then withdrawn, whereupon the scheme began to fold. The energy of its leader had gone. He had to be reinstated (Davis 1993, personal communication).

MENTAL HEALTH EDUCATION

In discussing mental health promotion, the Key Area Handbook (1993) concentrates mainly on preventive measures, but it does acknowledge that overall strategies must include an element which aims to increase awareness about mental illness and change public attitudes. The need is to: 'counter the fear, ignorance and stigma which still surround mental illness and create a more positive social climate in which it becomes more acceptable to talk about feelings, emotions and problems and to seek help without the fear of being labelled or feeling a failure.' This might be seen as the 'education' component of mental health promotion.

A group of psychiatric nurses in Derbyshire, working with elderly mentally ill people, set up a Mental Health Awareness Day to counter what they perceived as the hostility and ignorance shown to their unit by general hospital staff. They uncovered what they described as a 'hornet's nest' of unmet training needs, but also an enthusiasm for knowledge which was very encouraging (Nunn 1992). They have demonstrated what can be achieved by committed nurses working on their own initiative and with limited resources.

Until relatively recently, any practice nurse who wanted to include mental health issues in her health promotion campaigns would have had considerable difficulty in finding suitable posters and literature for patients. The Health Education Authority, who produce most of the health education materials used in primary care, have for years backed away from mental health. This may be about to change, but at the time of writing, they still produce little appropriate literature, except on alcohol (usually relating to its effects on physical health) and substance misuse.

Fortunately, there are other sources, not least the Defeat Depression Campaign jointly run by the Royal College of Psychiatrists and the Royal College of General Practitioners. One of the campaign's main objectives is to reduce the stigma associated with depression. It has now produced information leaflets and a book for the general public, guidelines and training packages for professionals and has plans for further developments.

A practice library

A librarian, Clare Pace (1992) has described a health education library set up in a surgery in Leeds. A review of the service showed mental health to be one of the most popular topics. The materials, which included books and audiotapes, were easily accessible so that patients could browse in the waiting room as well as borrow to read or listen at home. Worries that things would 'walk' proved largely unrealised, even though this was an urban practice. Health promotion units may be able to advise on similar schemes.

Consistency of messages is an important principle to establish when deciding on the kind of health education materials to use. Often, use is haphazard, and even professionals within the same practice may find themselves using different resources, sometimes giving conflicting information, as Lawson (1993) found during a survey undertaken in Northamptonshire. Patients and clients are quick to notice confusion and poor coordination. The result can all too easily undermine confidence and lead to rejection of the whole message.

Stress

In surveys, members of the general public commonly rate 'stress' as one of the major risk factors for coronary heart disease. Furthermore the other known risk factors – a diet high in saturated fat, smoking, high blood pressure, lack of exercise and family history – may be absent in up to 50% of all new cases (Niven 1989). This has led many health professionals to look at ways of helping their clients and patients reduce their stress. But stress affects more than physical health.

Sutherland and Cooper (1990) have shown that there may not only be effects on a wide range of physical illness, but social and work relationships and functioning as well. In all of these areas the negative effects of stress may be very costly.

In practical terms, helping people learn to handle stress better may be a useful way of promoting health, mental as well as physical. As an example, the Open University's 'Handling Stress' pack contains all that the experienced group leader needs to run a course. The materials concentrate on such issues as developing self-esteem, positive self-talk, enhancing social networks, assertiveness and coping skills, all of which might be said to protect against mental illness, specifically depression.

There are a number of other packs available which work along similar lines.

PSYCHOLOGICALLY-AWARE SUPPORT FOR STAFF

Traditionally, those who work in the caring professions have been expected to cope. To admit to difficulties was to risk being labelled ineffectual and to have 'black marks' against one's career. Many of today's practising nurses were, in training, actively discouraged from 'getting involved' with their patients' problems. This meant not only separating social life from work – which probably remains desirable – but also cultivating a 'hard' exterior which discouraged patients from attempting to discuss emotional problems with their nurse. It also meant that nurses who experienced an emotional crisis in their work – the death of a patient, for example, – were expected to be able to pick themselves up and carry on, using their own resources.

Such attitudes were always unrealistic. District nurses quickly learn that sharing patients' joys and griefs is part of the job. But the need for support for professional nurses in stressful situations has been slow to be recognised by employers. While a student health visitor some years ago the author was invited to join a support group set up by some health visiting colleagues with the help of a psychiatric social worker. Managers actively discouraged this initiative as time-wasting. In fact it proved an extremely valuable forum in which to discuss some of the very difficult issues health visitors often face.

Studies have shown that nurses who have high levels of social support with which they are well satisfied, report less stress and burn-out than others, regardless of the stress inherent in the job (Kellet 1991).

In a recent report, Millar (1994) outlines some current schemes, but says that only 1 in 10 health authorities and trusts have any written policy on staff support. She questions the morality of expecting staff to be sensitive to patients' needs whilst denying that they will have needs themselves.

It may seem obvious that occupational health departments should take a lead in providing support services, but they are mainly hospital-based and would still leave large numbers of community nurses, especially practice nurses, with no access.

Counsellors are expected to have on-going supervision from a suitably trained and experienced colleague throughout their professional lives. Nursing is at least as demanding and should develop a similar acceptance that support is an integral part of practice.

===================== CHAPTER NINE =====================

Meeting the targets

The *Health of the Nation* (1992) made a number of suggestions for ways in which primary care might make its contribution:

● Primary health care teams and local secondary care services will need to develop local good practice guidelines for the assessment and management of common psychiatric conditions, events and emergencies and for the use of the *Mental Health Act*.
● Training for primary care teams, . . . is necessary to help them improve their recognition and assessment of depression, anxiety and suicide risk, and to manage them appropriately.

The follow-up document 'First Steps' (1992) provided some more explicit ideas for purchasers, provider units, FHSAs and for primary care itself. Prominent among them, yet again, was the need for training to improve the 'recognition, assessment and management of depression, severe anxiety and suicide risk'.

Many more people are now being cared for in community settings rather than in hospital. Community care and primary care (which is also, of course, care outside hospital) are often seen by purchasers and commissioning agencies as being one and the same. This is misleading, as Figure 1.1 (page 2) has illustrated.

Primary care refers to the point of 'first contact' with the NHS for the patient or client, and is thus concerned mainly with:

(a) early detection and prompt treatment of illness;
(b) prevention of illness;
(c) promotion of health;
(d) management of chronic illness which either does not require hospital or specialist care, or is undertaken jointly with specialists.

The concept of community care means care outside hospital for people with established illness, disability or health needs. This is a step beyond 'first contact' and may therefore be seen as 'secondary care'. With numbers of FHSAs and DHAs joining together as Commissioning

Agencies the confusion surrounding these two terms becomes important, since primary care is in danger of losing out to the more high profile
and visible people with long-term mental illness. Patients are either psychotic and require expensive community care arrangements, or are
referred to disparagingly as the 'worried well' who shouldn't be
bothering the NHS.

Since at least 90% of people with psychiatric disorder are treated
within the primary care sector – by their GP – such attitudes are unrealistic and damaging. As Mann has pointed out (1992), research has
demonstrated few differences in the numbers and severity of symptoms
experienced by depressed people in hospital or GP settings.

Learning to cope more effectively with this morbidity is the main
contribution primary health care professionals can make to meeting the
Health of the Nation targets.

A ROLE FOR NURSES

The Department of Health has looked at nursing initiatives in the
Health of the Nation document 'Targeting Practice' (1993). Most of
the specific examples quoted in the Mental Illness Key Area relate to
secondary or hospital services, and although one (for mothers with
postnatal depression) has links with primary care, none are primary
care based.

One of the research projects mentioned is the KCW study which has
formed the basis of this book. Another, the Bath Model Practice
Project, which is running in parallel, has been overseen by a practice
nurse who has become a resource in mental health expertise for her
colleagues.

Health visitors in their work with families with young children are
clearly important not only in their ability to identify and help mothers
with postnatal depression, but also in the support they provide for young
families and in the teaching of good parenting skills.

District nurses, whose caseloads contain large numbers of people
with painful, disabling and life-threatening illness and who have regular
contact with their relatives and friends, are obviously in a position to
help some of those who are at high risk of becoming depressed.

A number of researchers (for example, Thomas & Corney 1993,
Wilkinson 1992b) are now focussing on the practice nurse as a key
person in identifying and providing care for depressed people in general
practice. A problem with some of this research is that it seems to be
based on a false premise – that practice nurses have plenty of time, and
that they need something to fill it.

The reality is that most practice nurses have no more time than their GP employers, and a not insubstantial proportion of them has been specifically employed to increase practice remuneration by concentrating on meeting income-generating targets such as cervical cytology and immunisation. Furthermore, the nursing press is continually bombarding them with exhortations about what they 'should' be doing for a wide variety of patients. Practice nurses are, above anything, generalists. In order to provide expert care, their need for knowledge and skills is almost limitless.

The 1992 census of practice nurses (Atkin & Lunt 1993) suggests that there are about 15 000 practice nursing posts nationwide. This is about 20% of all primary healthcare nurses. Half of these nurses have entered practice nursing since 1990, less than half have attended a practice nursing course and only about 13% have community nursing qualifications. There are apparently so few with the Registered Mental Nurse (RMN) qualification that it did not feature in the results at all.

In Thomas & Corney's (1993) survey, 89% of their practice nurse respondents said that they dealt with mental health problems – but 91% said they needed more training. It is the belief of these authors that mental health skills are an essential part of the repertoire of all health professionals. Paykel and Priest (1992) estimated that at least one patient with mild depression or worse would be present at each GP surgery session. If this is so for doctors, it is also likely to apply to practice nurses.

The framework which follows is an attempt by nurses themselves to describe the contribution they 'could' make to the care of people with depression and anxiety in primary care. It was compiled following a series of discussions and workshops with nurses involved in both the KCW study and the Bath Model Practice Project. They included practice nurses (two of whom specialise in mental health problems), a health visitor, a district nurse, a nurse practitioner who was also the practice counsellor and the KCW facilitator (Armstrong 1994).

As well as providing an outline of nursing interventions, the framework highlights the conditions under which this contribution could be made. These are vary far from being met. They include:

1. *Training*: a literature search into the mental health training needs of practice nurses, conducted by the Royal College of Nursing Library in 1991 for the author produced virtually nothing.
2. *Proper recognition*: of their professional status and responsibilities. There are two aspects to this: one is that nurses themselves must take their responsibilities seriously; but the other is that doctors need to understand that nurses are professionally accountable for their

actions. Many nurses complain that lack of this understanding leads to them being asked by employers to undertake tasks for which they are not trained.

3. *Good support*: without the support and agreement of the whole of the primary care team, practice nurses will not be able to develop the skills necessary to recognise and help people with psychological problems. FHSAs also need to recognise the support needs of this often very isolated group of nurses.

4. *Enough time*: there is a limit to how far the time allowed for individual appointments can be reduced without compromising quality of care. Many nurses find they are expected to complete a health check or well-woman examination (including a cervical smear) in only 10 minutes. This seems quite unrealistic.

The framework is described as a three-stage process. The stage at which any individual nurse is able to practice will depend on her level of skill, her interest in psychological problems, and the degree to which the above conditions apply.

Stage one

This is a baseline. All practice nurses who are RGN-qualified should have appropriate knowledge and skills to enable them to achieve this level of care.

In all the settings in which nurses offer health assessments, mental state should be assessed alongside other aspects. The guidelines in Figure 9.1 show how this might be achieved and the actions the nurse might need to take. Following such guidelines would help nurses in knowing when to refer potentially depressed people to the GP, and, by learning to elicit and list symptoms, to make credible referrals.

At Box 4, B meets the criteria for mild depression (as in Figure 3.2, Chapter 3). For these patients antidepressant therapy will not be appropriate, but there is still a need to recognise the distress. Social needs should be assessed and self-help advice offered. GP review may be necessary.

Patients who do not meet the criteria for mild depression may still have a range of problems and needs which require assessment. Referral to the practice counsellor (or external counselling service) may be acceptable. An extra appointment could be offered to any patient who would like more time.

Patients who fall into category C may have moderate to severe depression and should always be referred to the GP. Antidepressant

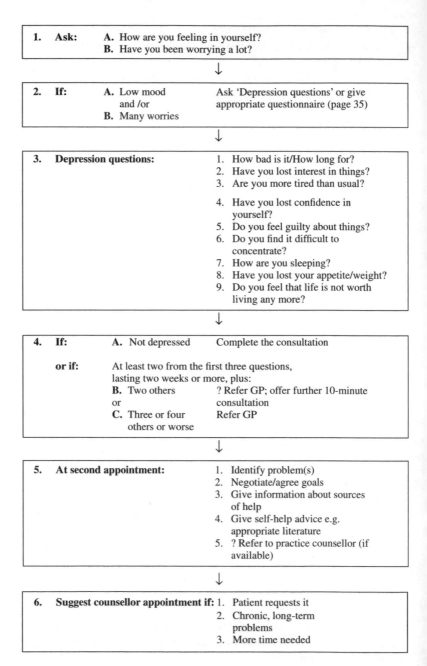

1.	**Ask:**	**A.** How are you feeling in yourself?
		B. Have you been worrying a lot?

↓

2.	**If:**	**A.** Low mood	Ask 'Depression questions' or give
		and /or	appropriate questionnaire (page 35)
		B. Many worries	

↓

3.	**Depression questions:**	1. How bad is it/How long for?
		2. Have you lost interest in things?
		3. Are you more tired than usual?
		4. Have you lost confidence in yourself?
		5. Do you feel guilty about things?
		6. Do you find it difficult to concentrate?
		7. How are you sleeping?
		8. Have you lost your appetite/weight?
		9. Do you feel that life is not worth living any more?

↓

4.	**If:**	**A.** Not depressed	Complete the consultation
	or if:	At least two from the first three questions, lasting two weeks or more, plus:	
		B. Two others	? Refer GP; offer further 10-minute
		or	consultation
		C. Three or four others or worse	Refer GP

↓

5.	**At second appointment:**	1. Identify problem(s)
		2. Negotiate/agree goals
		3. Give information about sources of help
		4. Give self-help advice e.g. appropriate literature
		5. ? Refer to practice counsellor (if available)

↓

6.	**Suggest counsellor appointment if:**	1. Patient requests it
		2. Chronic, long-term problems
		3. More time needed

Figure 9.1   *Guidelines for nurses*

medication may be indicated. Patients in categories B and C should be assessed for suicide risk (Chapter 3).

At a second appointment a problem-solving approach should be adopted. Referral to a counsellor might be suggested if:

1. the patient requests it;
2. there is evidence of chronic, long-term problems;
3. more time is needed.

These guidelines should not be implemented without thorough discussion within the practice, and the agreement of the whole primary care team. They could form the basis of a practice protocol.

Instead of the 'depression questions' an appropriate questionnaire such as the 12-point GHQ could be used.

In order to be able to use the guidelines, nurses will need:

- knowledge of depression and anxiety as they present in primary care; how to recognise symptoms; options for treatment (Chapters 3, 4 and 5);
- to be able to make an assessment of the patient's relevant social situation and provide information about local helping agencies (Chapters 4 and 7);
- to understand the role of the counsellor in primary care (Chapters 4 and 5);
- to be able to ask about suicide. An agreed practice protocol for helping patients who express suicidal thoughts or intentions is highly desirable (Chapters 3 and 7). Nurses should refer to the GP any patient who expresses suicidal ideas.

Stage two

Once all the above conditions are met, nurses might be in a position to extend their practice in one or more of the following ways:

1. Set up a programme of support and monitoring for people taking antidepressants in consultation with the GP. A minimum recommendation might be that patients on these drugs should be seen weekly for the first month, but not necessarily by the doctor. They should then be seen monthly for a further 4–6 months assuming progress is being made. Nurses could share this task using agreed guidelines such as those in Figure 9.2.
2. Incorporate mental health promotion into all general health promotion activities. This could be done by:
   (a) building an assessment of risk factors for depression into general health checks such as new patient checks and well-woman clinics;

At each appointment, check:	1. Compliance – is patient taking the medication?
	2. Dosage – is patient following the prescribed regime?
	3. Any side effects? Advice needed? If intolerable – refer GP
	4. Improvement? – reinforce continued treatment
	5. Deterioration? – refer GP

Figure 9.2   *Checking antidepressants*

   (b) setting up a practice library for patients;
   (c) using mental health related materials in surgery displays along-side other health information.
3. Set up a programme of liaison with local accident and emergency units to ensure that all people who attempt suicide get appropriate support. This might entail drawing up district-wide guidelines with colleagues from other practices, local managers, CPNs and social workers.
4. Provide straightforward advice and support for people who are tense, anxious and under stress such as explaining the mechanism of stress responses, relaxation training and stress diaries.
5. Evaluate nursing input.

Additional skills needed for practice at this stage would include:

- knowledge of commonly used antidepressants and their side-effects. A practice prescribing policy for these drugs will be desirable. Appropriate literature will be needed to provide information for patients about their medication (Chapter 4);
- knowledge of the risk factors for depression and suicide (Chapters 3 and 7);
- understanding of a problem-solving approach to reducing risk. Good interviewing and listening skills are essential (Chapter 7);
- understanding of and ability to use stress management techniques (Chapters 5 and 8);
- understanding of techniques for the management of severe anxiety and phobias including knowing where to obtain help for such patients in her area, for example clinical psychologists and CPNs (Chapter 5);

- understanding of clinical audit as it applies to general practice (Chapter 2 and Appendix).

Stage three

This is the stage for the nurse who wishes to specialise in the care of people with depression and anxiety in general practice. Notwithstanding the achievements of the practice nurse involved in the Model Practice Project (see below), or those taking part in what has become known as the Nurse Depression Study (Wilkinson *et al.* 1993), it is unlikely that nurses who do not have an RMN certificate would be able to obtain training so that they would be competent to practice at this level as things stand.

In addition to full implementation of Stage two, the nurse would:

1. In consultation with the GP, make full assessments of depressed people and manage care including follow-up of patients taking antidepressants (Wilkinson *et al.* 1993).
2. Maintain records of all 'high-risk' patients and ensure adequate support was available (Chapter 7).
3. Offer support to people wanting to withdraw from tranquilliser use (Russell & Lader 1993).
4. With GP support, develop the use of straightforward cognitive techniques for helping depressed and anxious people (France & Robson 1986).
5. In consultation with the GP, undertake audit of mental health related activities within the practice (Chapter 2).
6. Act as an adviser for other members of the practice team; support nursing colleagues.

As well as being a specialist within the practice, the nurse might also act as mentor to other interested practice nurses in her district. She would need at least the following additional skills and knowledge:

- clinical assessment of people with depression and anxiety;
- management of people with depression including monitoring of antidepressant therapy;
- counselling skills;
- knowledge of benzodiazepine withdrawal;
- cognitive-behavioural therapy.

The Bath Model Practice Project

(Information about this project has been supplied by Cathy Sutherland, Mental Health Focus Nurse.)

The project was set up in 1992, with funding from the Department of Health to run for 3 years in one GP practice. Another local practice acted as control. Evaluation methods were similar to those used in the KCW study. It was also a facilitation study, though in this case the facilitator was a member of the practice team, not an outside adviser.

The main aim of the project was to develop a system of care for people with mixed anxiety/depression, alcohol misuse, the elderly and the long-term mentally ill. The practice was far from being unique. It had the usual mix of doctors and nurses with varying attitudes, abilities and willingness to work with mentally ill people. Long-term objectives were to:

- Make mental illness an integral part of the everyday running of the practice.
- De-stigmatise depression for staff as well as patients.
- Create a transferable model to cascade 'good practice' nationwide.

The 'mental health focus nurse' was a general trained nurse, who, like most of her practice nurse colleagues, had no formal psychiatric nursing background. She was specially trained for this project. She provided educational input, support and resources to her fellow workers.

The nurses developed a system of 10–15 minute appointments during which they were able to recognise depressed people, arrange assessment using a short, structured interview, and refer for appropriate help. Referral might be to the doctor, the practice counsellor, community mental health team or a voluntary group for help with life difficulties. A Community Resource Book listed local agencies.

The nursing process was the basis of this approach. The nurse did not offer counselling. She began by agreeing a 'contract' with the patient, that although the interview was confidential, she would share information with the patient's doctor. This protected the nurse from having to cope alone with difficult disclosures and helped to avoid collusion.

There are several problems common to this and other projects, for instance:

1. Lack of teamwork. This may not be obvious at first, where the practice is regarded as a 'good' one, but there may be no common goals and no idea of working together to achieve them.
2. More fundamental, though perhaps related, may be the feeling among some nurses that they will do no more than absolutely necessary unless doctors are prepared to treat them as individual practitioners, and value their skills.

Sutherland describes the attitudes of two doctors:

- One took 'time out' to ask about nursing concerns, to discuss problems, debate solutions and boost confidence.
- Another was disruptive and made the nurse feel inferior. A great deal of patience and pain were needed to get to the stage where she felt that he had mellowed, and was easier to work with.

She illustrates the way in which she believes nurses can influence doctors using the story of a patient who was seen by the nurse for health promotion advice following a consultation with her GP.

The last thing this patient said as she left the nurse's room was 'I just feel so tired all the time'. Alarm bells rang and the nurse asked further questions, revealing a lady, caring for a terminally-ill husband, who felt she had come to the end of the road. The patient turned out to have been to the surgery every two weeks or so for about 11 months, with multiple physical symptoms. Numerous fruitless investigations had been carried out. A classic study in somatisation, who might have been recognised earlier.

At the time of writing, the Bath Project is continuing, and results are not yet available. The nature of the 'transferable model' is not yet clear. Nevertheless, the feeling on the ground is that care has improved, more depressed people are being recognised, and receiving treatment. As the project nurse points, out, we can reduce patients' suffering using relatively simple means even within the constraints of a 10 minute consultation.

CHALLENGES FOR THE FUTURE

The Bath Project and the framework described previously present a number of challenges: to nurses; to doctors; to educationalists; and to managers. Within each challenge there is a choice. Failure to meet the challenges constructively is likely to mean that primary care will fail to make its contribution to meeting the *Health of the Nation* targets. The challenges are :

- *To nurses*: The need for better mental health skills in primary care nurses is clearly demonstrated. Either nurses acquire the skills to meet the need or fail to provide comprehensive, quality health care for patients.
- *To doctors*: Nurses have a distinctive contribution to make to patient care. Either doctors recognise this and join nurses in developing a team approach to mental health care or continue to be swamped by the enormous demand. The demand will not go away.
- *To nurse educationalists*: Practice nurses need a repertoire of mental health skills. Help them acquire the skills through basic and

continuing education or nurses will look elsewhere for what they need. Quality will thus be variable and impossible to monitor.

- *To managers and purchasers*: Nurses need opportunities to update their skills, and they need support. Make the money and the time available to meet this need or risk the problems (legal and otherwise) which can arise if inadequately trained nurses undertake tasks for which they are ill-prepared, and risk increased sickness absence, high turnover and low morale where support is lacking.

The pay-off for primary care teams of improved mental health care is not that the health of the nation will improve. It is more immediate and self-interested than that.

Improving mental health care means that health care all round will improve. Patients will get better quicker.

And people who get better don't bother the doctor.

Auditing mental health care in general practice

This audit method was specially designed for the KCW FHSA Mental Health Facilitator Project (Chapter 2). The aims were:

- to provide feedback for the practices on the ability of the GPs to recognise depression since they were denied the results of the research evaluations;
- to provide information about the kind of care offered to people with high GHQ scores in the previous three months. This included consultation rate, mention in the records of a 'psychological' type diagnosis, concurrent physical illness, prescription and monitoring of psychotropic drugs, evidence of social assessment and type of referrals.

Although it was designed specially for the project, it has since been found useful elsewhere. It is given here as an example. It is not, of course, necessary to look at all the issues at one time. Practices wishing to audit mental health care may find it helpful to consult their local Medical Audit Advisory Group before they begin.

METHOD

Stage one

1. Approach 40 consecutive attenders in GP surgery. This number will give a statistically valid sample:

   (a) Choose patients in the age group 18–74.
   (b) Exclude private patients, temporary residents and any others whose care is atypical.
   (c) Use 'normal' surgery sessions, not special clinics.

2. Ask each patient to complete the 12-point Goldberg GHQ before going in to see the doctor (see Resources Section for details of how to obtain copies of this questionnaire). The GHQ is designed to identify patients who have a level of psychiatric illness ('cases'), not

simply people who are having a bad day. It does not diagnose depression.

Patients should, where possible, complete the questionnaire without assistance, though non-English speakers and anyone who admits to being unable to read could be helped. Excluding these people might give a false picture of the care being provided.

3. Ask the GP to score independantly each of these patients according to the following scale:

0 = no psychological symptoms present
1 = psychological symptoms are present

(The GP should not know the GHQ score before seeing the patient.)

The exercise can be done either practice-wide or by individual GP. A practice-wide audit avoids any suggestion of competition between partners, but there is likely to be a large variation in recognition which will not show up in a practice audit.

Scoring the GHQ

The GHQ has four columns of possible answers to the twelve questions. Each answer in the two left-hand columns scores 0; each answer in the two right-hand columns scores 1. To allocate the score, total the number of answers in the two right-hand columns. Researchers regard all patients scoring 2 or more as GHQ-positive. In practical terms this is probably too low, and you may prefer to use a score of 3 or 4. In general, increasing this threshold by 1 point reduces the number of positives by about 10%. People who score 4 or more probably have significant illness.

Add up the numbers of GHQ-positive patients (that is those scoring 3 or more, or whatever figure you decide to use as your threshold).

Identify how many of these patients have been scored '1' by the GP (that is, those who were recognised).

You can now calculate a measure of the GP's ability to recognise people with psychiatric illness:

Divide the number of GHQ-positive patients recognised, by the total number who were GHQ-positive. Multiply this by 100 to give a percentage. This is the 'recognition index'.

Stage two

1. Identify the records of all GHQ-positive patients. Mark them in some way to alert the GP at the next visit.

2. Using the records make a retrospective review of the care these patients have received in the previous three months:

(a) Number of consultations. Do not include special clinics.

(b) What is the main diagnosis? This may not be the reason for consultation. The aim is to note any major physical illness from which the patient is suffering.

(c) Is there any mention of a 'psychological' diagnosis in the previous three months. Note for instance depression, anxiety or other psychiatric illness. Also note words like distressed, worried, agitated, tense, disturbed and so on.

(d) Has the patient received, or is he/she currently receiving any psychotropic medication? Note antidepressants, anxiolytics, for example valium and hypnotics.

(e) Write down dosage and regime.

(f) Note whether there are arrangements to monitor the prescription and the patient. If your practice has a protocol, this will be obvious, otherwise note mention of side-effects and advice on minimising these.

(g) Has any assessment of social difficulties been made in the previous three months? Clues to this would be mention of the patient's domestic situation: for example, career, financial difficulties, marital problems, worries about family.

(h) Has any referral been made? Include referral to hospital for investigations of physical symptoms and also to practice counsellor, psychiatric units, social services, self-help group or other helping agency.

What to do with the results

From the results it is possible to answer certain questions about the mental health care offered in your practice:

- Do frequent attenders have high GHQ scores? Are they known to have psychological or social difficulties? Do they need further assessment or help?

- Are there people with serious physical illness whose mental state has not been assessed? Are any of these people suffering from depression which requires treatment?

- How often is a psychological assessment made alongside a physical examination?

- What are your criteria for prescribing antidepressants and/or benzodiazepines? Are antidepressant given in therapeutic dose for an adequate length of time, and are they monitored?

- For how many of these people has a social assessment been made?
- To whom do you refer most often? Do you need to improve your knowledge of local sources of help for people with psychological and social difficulties?

The answers to these questions can be used in a variety of ways:

- To assess actual care against a previously agreed standard.
- To provide a baseline against which improvements can be measured.
- To identify points at which change may be required.

Stage three

Repeat audit – 6 months later

1. Review again the care of these same patients:
   Has the consultation rate changed?
   Are any still taking psychotropic medication?
2. Repeat audit from Stage one reviewing the care of a new set of patients.

Equipment needed

1. 40 copies of the 12-point General Health Questionnaire. (Other suitable questionnaires could be used, adjusting the method of calculation appropriately.) 2 clip-boards and pens.
2. 40 copies of letters inviting patients to take part in your 'stress' survey, on practice headed note-paper.
3. Copies of suitable forms on which to record findings.
4. Copies of letters for GPs explaining what you are asking them to do (especially if you are an outside facilitator conducting the audit).

Adams, A. (1992) *Bullying at Work. How to Confront and Overcome it.* London, Virago.

Alderman, C. (1993) Keeping on the Right Track. *Nursing Standard*, 7(21): 18–19.

Allsop, J. (1990) *Changing Primary Care: The Role of Facilitators.* London, Kings Fund Centre.

Armstrong, E. (1993a) Mental Health Check. *Nursing Times*, 89(33): 40–42.

Armstrong, E. (1993b) Mental Health Promotion. In Dines, A. & Cribb, A. (Eds) *Health Promotion: Concepts and Practice.* London, Blackwell Scientific Publications.

Armstrong, E. (1994) A Framework for Depression. *Practice Nurse*, 15–31 May. 516–520.

Atkin, K. & Lunt, N. (1993) Nurses Count – First National Census. *Practice Nurse*, 15–31 Oct. 593–598.

BAC (1990) Code of Ethics and Practice for Counsellors. British Association for Counselling.

BAC (1993) Counselling in Medical Settings. Guidelines for the Employment of Counsellors in General Practice. British Association For Counselling.

Barbee, A.P. (1990) Interactive Coping: The Cheering-up Process in Close Relationships. In Duck, S. (Ed) *Personal Relationships and Social Support.* London, Sage Publications.

Bayley R. (1993) Hear our Voices. *Nursing Times*, 89(25): 32–33.

Berg, J.H. & Piner, K. (1990) Social Relationships and the Lack of Social Relationships. In Duck, S. (Ed) *Personal Relationships and Social Support.* London, Sage Publications.

Blacker, C.V.R. & Clare, A.W. (1987) Depressive Disorder in Primary Care. *British Journal of Psychiatry*, 150: 737–751.

Braithwaite, R. (1992) *Violence: Understanding, Intervention and Prevention.* Oxford, Radcliffe Professional Press.

Briscoe, M. (1989) The Detection of Emotional Disorders in the Postnatal Period by Health Visitors. *Health Visitor*, 62: 336–338.

Brown, G.W. (1992) Life Events and Social Support: Possibilities for Primary Prevention. In Jenkins, R., Newton, J. & Young, R. *The Prevention of Depression and Anxiety: The Role of the Primary Care Team.* London, HMSO.

Brown, G.W. & Harris, T.O. (1978) *Social Origins of Depression.* London, Tavistock.

Burke, M. (1992) Counselling in General Practice, Options for Action: a Social Worker's Point of View. In Jenkins, R., Newton, J. and Young, R. (Eds) *The*

Prevention of Depression and Anxiety: The Role of the Primary Care Team. London, HMSO.

Care Programme Approach for People with a Mental Illness Referred to the Specialist Psychiatric Services, The. (1990) Joint Health and Social Services circular HC(90)23/LASSL(90)11. London, Department of Health.

Casey, P. (1993) *A Guide to Psychiatry in Primary Care.* Petersfield, Wrightson Biomedical Publishing Ltd.

CETHV (1977) An Investigation into the Principles of Health Visiting. London, Council for the Education and Training of Health Visitors.

Childs-Clarke, A., Whitfield, W., Cadbury, S. and Sandu, S. (1989) Anxiety Management Groups in Clinical Practice. *Nursing Times*, 85(30): 49–52.

Clinical Psychology and General Practice (1991). In *Drugs and Therapeutics Bulletin*, 29(3): 9–11. Consumers Association.

Cockburn, J., Ruth, D., Silagy, C., Dobbin, M., Reid, Y., Scollo, M. & Naccarella, L. (1992) Randomised Trial of Three Approaches of Marketing Smoking Cessation Programmes to Australian General Practitioners. *BMJ*. 304: 691–694.

Code of Professional Conduct for the Nurse, Midwife and Health Visitor (1992). London, UKCC.

Corney, R. (1992a) The Effectiveness of Counselling in General Practice. *International Review of Psychiatry*, 4: 331–338.

Corney, R. (1992b) Evaluation of the Effectiveness of Counselling. In Sheldon, M. (Ed) *Counselling in General Practice.* London, Royal College of General Practitioners.

Corney, R. & Jenkins, R. (1993) Counselling in General Practice Today. In Corney, R. & Jenkins, R. *Counselling in General Practice.* London, Routledge.

Corob, A. (1987) *Working with Depressed Women: a Feminist Approach.* Aldershot, Gower Publishing Company Ltd.

Cox, J.L., Holden, J.M. & Sagovsky, R. (1987) Detection of Postnatal Depression, Development of the 10-item Edinburgh Postnatal Depression Scale. *British Journal of Psychiatry*, 150: 782–786.

Coyle, J., Calnan, M., & Williams, S. (1993) Changing Perceptions. *Nursing Times*, 89(25): 44–46.

Crammer, J. & Heine, B. (1991) *The Use of Drugs in Psychiatry.* London, Gaskell/Royal College of Psychiatrists.

Dietrich, A.J., O'Connor, G.T., Keller, A., Carney, P.A., Levy, D. & Whaley, F.S. (1992) Cancer: Improving Early Detection and Prevention. A Community Practice Randomised Trial. *BMJ*, 304: 687–691.

Dines, A. & Cribb, A. (1993) (Eds) *Health Promotion: Concepts and Practice.* London, Blackwell Scientific Publications.

Effective Health Care, Bulletin 5. (1993) The Treatment of Depression in Primary Care. School of Public Health. Leeds University.

Essex, B., Doig, R. & Renshaw, J. (1990) Pilot Study of Records of Shared Care for People with Mental Illnesses. *BMJ*, 33: 1442–6.

Evans, M. (1993) Suicide: a Target for Health. RCN Nursing Update. *Nursing Standard*, 7(18): 9–14.

Fernando, S. (1993) Combating Racism in Mental Health Services. *Open Mind*, 61: 18–19.

France, R. & Robson, M. (1986) *Behaviour Therapy in Primary Care: a Practical Guide.* Kent, Croom Helm.

Fullard, E., Fowler, G. & Gray, M. (1984) Facilitating Prevention in Primary Care. *BMJ*, 289: 1585–1587.

Fullard, E., Fowler, G. & Gray, M. (1987) Promoting Prevention in Primary Care: Controlled Trial of Low Technology, Low Cost Approach. *BMJ*, 294: 1080–1082.

Gask, L. (1992) Teaching Psychiatric Interview Skills to General Practitioners. In Jenkins, R., Newton, J. & Young, R. (Eds) *The Prevention of Depression and Anxiety: The Role of the Primary Care Team.* London, HMSO.

Goldberg, D. & Huxley, P. (1980) *Mental Illness in the Community: The Pathway to Psychiatric Care.* London, Tavistock.

Goldberg, D., Bridges, K., Duncan-Jones, P. and Grayson, D. (1988) Detecting Anxiety and Depression in General Medical Settings. *BMJ*, 297: 8 Oct. 897–899.

Goldberg, D. & Williams, P. (1988) *A User's Guide to the GHQ.* London, NFER-Nelson.

Goldberg, D. (1992) Early Diagnosis and Secondary Prevention. In Jenkins, R., Newton, J. & Young, R. (Eds) *The Prevention of Depression and Anxiety: The Role of the Primary Care Team.* London, HMSO.

Grieves, R. (1993) The Effects of Physical Illness. *Practice Nursing*, 16 Mar–5 Apr. 16.

Hammersley, D. & Beeley, L. (1992) The Effects of Medication on Counselling. *Counselling*, 3(3): 162–164.

Health of the Nation, The. (1992) *A Strategy for Health in England.* London, HMSO.

Health of the Nation, The. (1992) *First Steps for the NHS.* London, NHS Management Executive.

Health of the Nation, The. (1993) *Key Area Handbook – Mental Illness.* London, Department of Health.

Health of the Nation, The. (1993) *Targeting Practice: The Contribution of Nurses, Midwives and Health Visitors.* London, Department of Health.

Hill, D. (1993) Psychiatry's Lost Cause. *Open Mind*, 61: 18–19.

Holden, J.M., Sagovsky, R. & Cox, J.L. (1989) Counselling in a General Practice Setting: Controlled Study of Health Visitor Intervention in Treatment of Postnatal Depression. *BMJ*, 298: 223–226.

Howard, A. (1992) What, and Why are we Accrediting? *Counselling*, 3(3): 171–173.

Howson, R. (1991) Look After your Heart/ Look After Yourself: for People with Special Needs. South Durham Health Care. Unpublished.

Jenkins, R. & Shepherd, M. (1983) Mental Illness and General Practice. In Bean, P. (Ed) *Mental Illness, Changes and Trends.* London, John Wiley and Sons Ltd.

Jenkins, R. (1992a) A Multiaxial Approach to the Primary Care of Schizophrenia. In Jenkins, R., Field, V. and Young, R. (Eds) *The Primary Care of Schizophrenia.* London, HMSO.

Jenkins, R., (1992b) Developments in the Primary Care of Mental Illness – a Forward Look. *International Review of Psychiatry*, 4: 237–242.

Jenkins, R. (1992c) Depression and Anxiety: An Overview of Preventive Strategies . In Jenkins, R., Newton, J. & Young, R. (Eds) *The Prevention of Depression and Anxiety: the Role of the Primary Care Team.* London, HMSO.

Kellett, J. (1991) Caring About Each Other. *Nursing Standard*, 5(48): 46.

Kiernan, P. (1992) Counselling in General Practice: an Evaluation of the Work of GP and Counsellor. Unpublished personal communication.

King, M.B., Gabe, J., Williams, P. and Rodrigo, K. (1990) Long-term use of Benzodiazepines: the Views of Patients. *Brit. J. Gen. Pract.* 40: 194–196.

King, M.B. (1993) Is There Still a Role for Benzodiazepines in General Practice? *Brit. J. Gen. Pract.* 42: 202–205.

Lacey, R. (1991) *The Complete Guide to Psychiatric Drugs.* London, Ebury Press/MIND.

Lader, M. (1989) Benzodiazepines in Profile. *Prescribers Journal*, 29: 1, 12–17.

Lawrie, S. (1993) Recognising the Features and Making a Diagnosis in Schizophrenia: Approaches to Diagnosis and Therapy. *Prescriber*, 19 Feb. 41–45.

Lawson, L. (1993) It's a Bit like Wallpaper! Survey into Use of Health Promotion Literature in Primary Care. Unpublished personal communication.

Leff, J. (1992) Schizophrenia: Aetiology, Prognosis and Course. In Jenkins, R., Field, V. & Young, R. (Eds) *The Primary Care of Schizophrenia.* HMSO, London.

Livingston, M. (1990) Tricyclic and Newer Antidepressants. *Prescribers Journal*, 30(4): 139–147.

Lloyd, K. (1992) Ethnicity, Primary Care and Non-psychotic Disorders. *International Review of Psychiatry*, 4: 257–265.

Mann, A. (1992) Depression and Anxiety in Primary Care: The Epidemiological Evidence. In Jenkins, R., Newton, J. & Young, R. (Eds) *The Prevention of Depression and Anxiety: the Role of the Primary Care Team.* London, HMSO.

Mann, A.H, Jenkins, R. & Belsey, E. (1981) The Twelve-month Outcome of Patients with Neurotic Illness in General Practice. *Psychological Medicine*, 11: 535–550.

Mann, A. & Jenkins, R. (1982) The Outcome of Neurotic Illness in General Practice. *Update*, 15 Jul. 254–261.

Mares, P., Henley, A. & Baxter, C. (1985) *Health Care in Multi-racial Britain.* London, Health Education Council/National Extension College.

Marsh, G.N. (1993) The Counsellor as Part of the General Practice Team. In Corney, R. & Jenkins, R. (Eds) *Counselling in General Practice.* London, Routledge.

Maxwell, H. (Ed) (1990) *Psychotherapy: an Outline for Medical Students and Practitioners.* London, Whurr Publishers Ltd.

McLeod, J. (1992) The General Practitioner's Role. In Sheldon, M. (Ed) *Counselling in General Practice.* London, RCGP.

Mead, M. (1992) Drugs for Depression and Anxiety. *Practice Nurse*, Oct. 382–387.

Millar, B. (1994) Listen Very Carefully. *Health Service Journal*, 20 Jan. 10–11.

MORI (1992) Attitudes Towards Depression: Research Study for the Defeat Depression Campaign. London, Royal College of Psychiatrists.

Morrell, V. (1992) Developing Counselling Skills. In Sheldon, M. (Ed) *Counselling in General Practice.* London, RCGP.

Mortimer, A. (1993) Organising Appropriate Drug Regimens in Schizophrenia: Approaches to Diagnosis and Therapy. *Prescriber*, 19 Feb. 46–52.

Mumford, D.B., Bavington, J.T., Bhatnagar, K.S., Hussein, Y., Mirza, S. & Naraghi, M.M. (1991) The Bradford Somatic Inventory: A Multi-ethnic

Inventory of Somatic Symptoms Reported by Anxious and Depressed Patients in Britain and the Indo-Pakistan Subcontinent. *British Journal of Psychiatry,* 158: 379–386.

Murray, R.M. (1993) Biologically Vulnerable. *Open Mind,* 61: 14–15.

Murray, R., Hurle, D. and Grant, A. (1991) Tranquillisers: *The MIND Guide to Where to Get Help.* MIND Publications/University of Bradford.

Nelson-Jones, R. (1991) *Practical Counselling and Helping Skills.* London, Cassell.

Newton, J. (1988) *Preventing Mental Illness.* London, Routledge.

Newton, J. (1992a) *Preventing Mental Illness in Practice.* London, Routledge.

Newton, J. (1992b) Crisis Support: Utilising Resources. In Jenkins, R., Newton, J. & Young, R. (Eds) *The Prevention of Depression and Anxiety: The Role of the Primary Care Team.* London, HMSO.

Niven, N. (1989) *Health Psychology. An Introduction for Nurses and Other Health Care Professionals.* Edinburgh, Churchill Livingstone.

Nunn, D. (1992) Inside the Hornet's Nest. *Nursing the Elderly,* 4(6): 16–17.

Pace, C. (1992) Health Information: A Health Education Library in General Practice. In Jenkins, R., Newton, J. and Young, R. (Eds) *The Prevention of Depression and Anxiety: The Role of the Primary Care Team.* London, HMSO.

Parkes, C.M. (1986) *Bereavement: Studies of Grief in Adult Life.* London, Penguin Books.

Paykel, E.S. & Priest, R.G. (1992) Recognition and Management of Depression in General Practice: Consensus Statement. *BMJ,* 305: 1198–1202.

Pringle, M., Bilkhu, J., Dornan, M. & Head, S. (1991) *Managing Change in Primary Care.* Oxford, Radcliffe Medical Press.

Pritchard, P. & Pritchard, J. (1992) *Developing Teamwork in Primary Health Care: A Practical Workbook.* Oxford, Oxford University Press.

Report of the Enquiry into London's Health Service, Medical Education and Research. (Tomlinson Report) (1992) London, HMSO.

Robinson, G., Beaton, S. & White, P. (1993) Attitudes Towards Practice Nurses – Survey of a Sample of General Practitioners in England and Wales. *Brit. J. Gen. Pract.* 43: 25–29.

Rowe, D. (1983) Depression: *The Way out of Your Prison.* London, Routledge and Kegan Paul.

Rowland, N. (1992) Counselling and Counselling Skills. In Sheldon, M. (Ed) *Counselling in General Practice.* London, RCGP.

Royal College of General Practitioners (1981) Prevention of Arterial Disease in General Practice, Report from General Practice 19. London, RCGP.

Royal College of General Practitioners (1981) Prevention of Psychiatric Disorders in General Practice. Report from General Practice 20. London, RCGP.

Ruddy, B. (1992) Brief Encounters. *Health Service Journal,* 17 Sept. 22–24.

Rushton, A. and Briscoe, M. (1981) Social Work as an Aspect of Primary Care: The Social Workers' View. *Br. J. Social Wk,* 11: 61–76.

Russell, G. & Hersov, L. (1983) *Handbook of Psychiatry,* 4: 205–206. Cambridge University Press.

Russell, J. and Lader, M. (1993) *Guidelines for the Prevention and Treatment of Benzodiazepine Dependence.* Mental Health Foundation.

Sartorius, N. (1992) The Promotion of Mental Health: Meaning and Tasks. In Trent, D.R. (Ed) *Promotion of Mental Health,* Vol. 1. Aldershot, Avebury.

Shah, A. (1992) The Burden of Psychiatric Disorder in Primary Care. *International Review of Psychiatry*, 4: 243–250.

Sharp, D. (1992) Liaison between Providers of Primary Care: Early Detection Difficulties. B. Predicting Postnatal Depression. In Jenkins, R., Newton, J. & Young, R. (Eds) *The Prevention of Depression and Anxiety: the Role of the Primary Care Team*. London, HMSO.

Sheldon, T.A., Freemantle, N., House, A., Adams, C.E., Mason, J.M., Song, F., Long, A. & Watson, P. (1993) Examining the Effectiveness of Treatments for Depression in General Practice. *Journal of Mental Health*, 2: 141–156.

Shepherd, G. (1992) The Management of Schizophrenia in the Community: What Services do we Need? In Jenkins, R., Field, V. & Young, R. (Eds) *The Primary Care of Schizophrenia*. London, HMSO.

Sims, A. (1993) The Scar that is More than Skin Deep: the Stigma of Depression. *Brit. J. Gen. Pract.* 43: 30–31.

Spiegal, N., Murphy, E., Kinmoth, A-L., Ross, F., Bain, J. & Coates, R. (1992) Managing Change in General Practice: a Step-by-step Guide. *BMJ*, 304: 231–234.

Standardised Assessment Scales for Elderly People (1992). Report of Joint Workshops of the Research Unit of the Royal College of Physicians and the British Geriatrics Society, London.

Sutherland, V.J. and Cooper, C. (1990) *Understanding Stress: a Psychological Perspective for Health Professionals*. London, Chapman and Hall.

Tantam, D. (1992) Schizophrenia: What Treatment is Available? In Jenkins, R., Field, V. & Young, R. (Eds) *The Primary Care of Schizophrenia*. London, HMSO.

Thomas, R.V.R. & Corney, R.H. (1992) A Survey of Links Between Mental Health Professionals and General Practice in Six Health Authorities. *Brit. J. Gen. Pract.* 42: 358–361.

Thomas, R.V.R. & Corney, R.H. (1993) The Role of the Practice Nurse in Mental Health: A Survey. *Journal of Mental Health*, 2: 65–72.

Tolley, K. (1993) *Health Promotion: How to Measure Cost Effectiveness*. London, Health Education Authority.

Tovet, R. (1992) Linking with Voluntary and Community Resources: Camden Tranquilliser Services. In Jenkins, R., Newton, J. and Young, R. (Eds) *The Prevention of Depression and Anxiety: The Role of the Primary Care Team*. London, HMSO.

Torkington, N.P.K. (1991) *Black Health: a Political Issue*.Liverpool, Catholic Association for Racial Justice/Liverpool Institute of Higher Education.

Tredgold, R.F. & Wolff, H.H. (1984) (Eds) *UCH Handbook of Psychiatry*. London, Duckworth.

Trent, D.R. (1991) Breaking the Single Continuum. In Trent D.R. (Ed) *Promotion of Mental Health*, Vol. 1. Aldershot, Avebury.

Trent, D.R. (1993) The Promotion of Mental Health: Fallacies of Current Thinking. In Trent, D.R. & Reed, C. (Eds) *Promotion of Mental Health*, Vol. 2. Aldershot, Avebury.

Turner, G. (1993) Client/CPN Contact During Administration of Depot Medications: Implications for Practice. In Brooker, C. & White, E. (Eds) *Community Psychiatric Nursing: A Research Perspective*, Vol. 2. London, Chapman & Hall.

Turner, T.H. (1986) Whatever Happened to Stigma? *Bulletin of RCPsych.* 10: 8–9, London.

Tylee, A. & Freeling, P (1988) Sensitizing to a Diagnosis of Depression. *Horizons*, May, 269–276.

Usherwood, V. (1993a) Depression: Lifting the Cloud. RCN Nursing Update. *Nursing Standard*, 7(18): 3–8.

Usherwood, V. (1993b) Problem Based Interviewing, *Practice Nursing*, 2–15 Feb.

van de Kar, A., Knotterus, A., Meertens, R., Dubois, V. & Kok, G. (1992) Why Do Patients Consult their General Practitioner? Determinants of their Decision. *Brit. J. Gen. Pract.* 42: 313–316.

Warner, R.W., Gater, R., Jackson, M.G. & Goldberg, D.P. (1993) Effects of a Community Mental Health Service on the Practice and Attitudes of General Practitioners. *Brit. J. Gen. Pract.* 43: 507–511.

Wilkinson, D.G. (1989) *Depression: Recognition and Treatment in General Practice.* Oxford, Radcliffe Medical Press.

Wilkinson, G. (1992a) *Anxiety: Recognition and Treatment in General Practice.* Oxford, Radcliffe Medical Press.

Wilkinson, G. (1992b) The Role of the Practice Nurse in the Management of Depression. *International Review of Psychiatry*, 4: 311–316.

Wilkinson, G., Allen, P., Marshall, E., Walker, J., Browne, W. & Mann, A.H. (1993) The Role of the Practice Nurse in the Management of Depression in General Practice: Treatment Adherence to Antidepressant Medication. *Psychological Medicine*, 23: 229–237.

Wilkinson, M.J.B. and Barczak, P. (1988) Psychiatric Screening in General Practice – Comparison of the GHQ and the HAD Scale. *JRCollGP*, Jul. 311–313.

Williams, J.M.G. & Pollock, L. (1993) Factors Mediating Suicidal Behaviour: Their Utility in Primary and Secondary Prevention. *Journal of Mental Health*, 2: 3–26.

Williams, R. (1993) Psychiatric Morbidity in Children and Adolescents: a Suitable Cause for Concern. *Brit. J. Gen. Pract.* 43: 3–4.

Wright, A. (1988) *Depression: A Major Problem in General Practice.* London, Royal College of General Practitioners.

Wright, A.F. (1993) *Depression: Recognition and Management in General Practice.* London, RCGP.

ESSENTIAL READING

Jenkins, R., Newton, J. & Young, R. (Eds) (1992) *The Prevention of Anxiety and Depression. The Role of the Primary Care Team.* London, HMSO.
Jenkins, R., Field, V. & Young, R. (Eds) (1992) *The Primary Care of Schizophrenia.* London, HMSO.
Wilkinson, D.G. (1989) *Depression: Recognition and Treatment in General Practice.* Oxford, Radcliffe Medical Press.
Wilkinson, G. (1992) *Anxiety: Recognition and Treatment in General Practice.* Oxford, Radcliffe Medical Press.
Pritchard, P. & Pritchard, J. (1992) *Developing Teamwork in Primary Health Care: A Practical Workbook.* Oxford, Oxford University Press.

QUESTIONNAIRES AND RATING SCALES

For copies of the 12-point General Health Questionnaire and the HAD Scale contact:

NFER-Nelson Publishing Co. Ltd
Darville House
2 Oxford Road East
Windsor
Berks SL4 1BU

For details of the Edinburgh Postnatal Depression Scale see Cox *et al.* (1987) (References list).

For the Beck Depression Inventory see France & Robson (1986) (References list).

Information about these scales is also available from the Defeat Depression Campaign.

USEFUL ADDRESSES

National Facilitator Development Project
HEA Primary Health Care Unit
Block 10
Churchill Hospital
Headington
Oxford OX3 7LJ   Tel: 01865 226052/3

Details of the Association of Primary Care Facilitators can be obtained from the above office.

Defeat Depression Campaign
Royal College of Psychiatrists
17 Belgrave Square
London SW1X 8PG   Tel: 0171 235 2351

(variety of leaflets for patients, training package for GPs and other materials: send SAE for samples; also factsheets on aspects of mental illness including the Mental Health Act)

British Association for Counselling
(including Counselling in Medical Settings Division)
1 Regent Place
Rugby CV21 2PJ   Information line: 01788 578328

(information on all aspects of counselling; directory of counsellors and training organisations; guidelines for the employment of counsellors in general practice)

Counselling in Primary Care Trust
Suite 3a
Majestic House
High Street
Staines TW18 4DG   Tel: 01784 442601

(research database on counselling in primary care and other information; training for counsellors who want to work in primary care)

Mental Health Foundation
37 Mortimer Street
London W1N 7RJ   Tel: 0171 580 0145

(leaflets for patients on mental health subjects and booklet 'Guidelines for the prevention and treatment of benzodiazepine dependence')

MIND
Granta House
15–19 Broadway
Stratford
London E15 4BQ   Tel: 0181 519 2122

(variety of information sheets and booklets for users; local groups and other publications).

Samaritans
(National Office)
10 The Grove
Slough
Berks SL1 1QP   Tel: 01753 532713
(see Phone Book for your local office)

PROFESSIONAL EDUCATION

For GPs: Contact the Defeat Depression campaign or your Regional Tutor for details of training package.

For nurses: RCN Nursing Update have produced two learning units:

Depression: Lifting the cloud
Suicide: A target for health
(In preparation: Counselling Skills)
Telephone Royal College of Nursing: 0171 409 3333 for details of your nearest viewing centre.

For primary care teams: A course in primary mental health care for primary care teams is being piloted. For details, contact:

Royal Institute of Public Health and Hygiene
28 Portland Place
London W1N 4DE   Tel: 0171 580 2731

Handling stress: A teaching pack is produced by the Open University containing everything needed by an experienced group leader to run a course on Handling Stress. For details, contact:

Central Enquiry Service
PO Box 200
The Open University
Walton Hall
Milton Keynes MK7 6AA

FOR YOUR PRACTICE LIBRARY

1. Books

The Complete Guide to Psychiatric Drugs: A Layman's Handbook by Ron Lacey. Published by MIND and Ebury Press.

Tranquillisers: the MIND Guide to Where to Get Help by Murray, Hurle and Grant. Published by MIND.

MIND publications are available from: MIND Mail Order Service, 4th Floor, 24–32 Stephenson Way, London NW1 2HD. Tel: 0171 387 9126

Depression: The Way Out of Your Prison by Dorothy Rowe.
Published by Routledge.

Self-help for Your Nerves by Dr Claire Weekes. Published by Fontana.
(This book was first published in 1962, but continues to be very popular and is regularly reprinted. The author has written a number of other self-help books for patients.)

Down with Gloom! by Brice Pitt with cartoons by Mel Calman. Published by the Defeat Depression Campaign.

The above books are available in bookshops.

See also the 'Overcoming Common Problems' series. Details from: Sheldon Press, Holy Trinity Church, Marylebone Road, London NW1 4DU.
Tel: 0171 387 5282.

2. Audiotapes

Anxiety and stress management:

Lifeskills
Bowman House
6 Billetfield
Taunton TA1 3NN

Relaxation for Living
168-170 Oaklands Drive
Weybridge
Surrey KT13 9ET

Mental health problems:
National Schizophrenia Fellowship
28 Castle Street
Kingston on Thames
Surrey KT1 1SS
Tel: 0181 547 3937

Pax (Tapes for sufferers from panic attacks, phobias and anxiety disorders)
4 Manorbrook
Blackheath
London SE3 9AW

OTHER SOURCES OF INFORMATION

The BBC Family Directory available in bookshops or direct from:

Health Education Authority
Hamilton House
Mabledon Place
London WC1H 9TX
Tel: 0171 413 1946

Help for Health Trust
Tel: 01962 848100
(Database of over 3000 organisations)

The Defeat Depression Campaign has lists of national self-help organisations.

Contact-a-Family produces a directory of self-help and support groups for parents of children who suffer from every imaginable syndrome, however rare. Their address is:
16 Strutton Ground
London SW1P 2HP
Tel: 0171 222 2695

Benefits For up-to-date copies of leaflets and posters on benefits, join the Benefits Agency Publicity Register. Tel: 01645 540000.

For local information see your Phone Book or contact your practice health visitor or district nurse, Social Services department, Council for Voluntary Service, Citizen's Advice Bureau or the public library.

TIPS FOR COMPILING A LOCAL DIRECTORY

When compiling a directory for use in general practice settings, the following ideas have proved useful:

1. Use common problems as headings. This facilitates problem-solving.

   Suggested headings are:
   bereavement; couples/relationships/psychosexual; parents and children; other family problems; support for carers; physical illness/disability; psychiatric illness; debt/housing/legal.

Work-related problems:
redundancy/unemployment/discrimination/bullying.

2. Include major national organisations as sources of information, but concentrate on local groups for practical help and support.

3. Your local Health Promotion Unit or FHSA might be able to help produce and maintain a local directory. Reminder cards containing the phone numbers of a few key local agencies – those that you use most – may be usefully kept on your desk.

4. Consider asking your local Health Promotion Unit to design a problem-solving booklet for patients and clients which could be available in the practice waiting room or library. This would be quite simple to produce using desk-top publishing software.

5. Keep your register up to date. Even major national charities move!